SEXUAL HAPPINESS FOR MEN
A Practical Approach

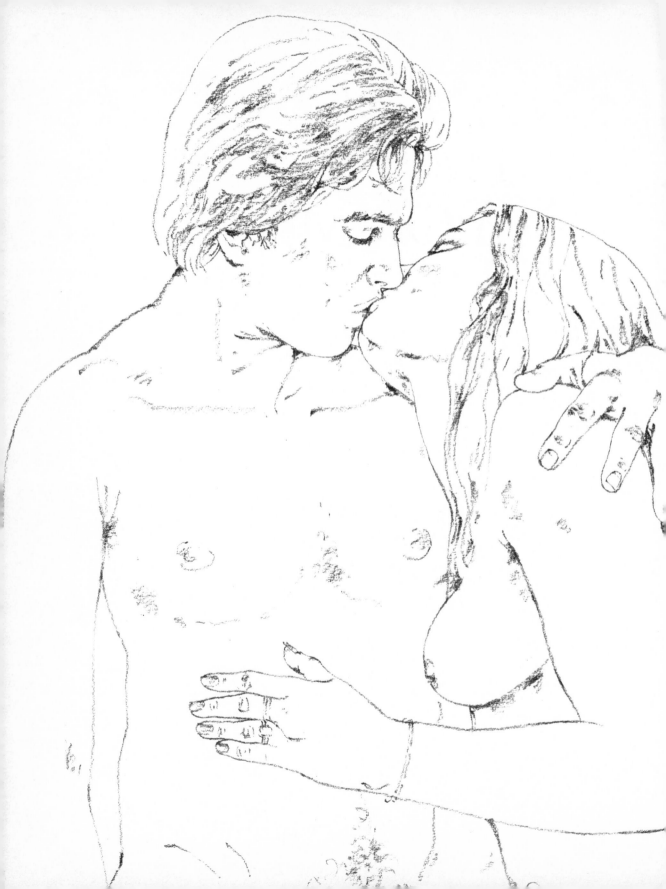

SEXUAL HAPPINESS FOR MEN
A Practical Approach

MAURICE YAFFÉ

Senior Clinical Psychologist,
York Clinic, Guy's Hospital, London

ELIZABETH FENWICK

CONSULTANT EDITORS

RAYMOND C. ROSEN, Ph.D.

Associate Professor of Psychiatry,
Rutgers Medical School, New Jersey

JOHN M. KELLETT

Consultant Psychiatrist and Senior Lecturer,
St. George's Hospital Medical School, London

Illustrated by
Charles Raymond

An Owl Book

HENRY HOLT AND COMPANY
NEW YORK

Sadly, my friend and colleague Maurice Yaffé died shortly before we were to begin revising Sexual Happiness. *Maurice's kindness and his enthusiasm for any project he was involved in made him always a delightful and rewarding person to work with. He was also a skilled therapist whose wide experience of people and their sexual problems was an incalculable help to me in writing the book.*

I am very grateful to Dr. John Kellett for collaborating with me on this new edition.
E. F.

Editor Richard Dawes
Art editor Philip Lord
Assistant designer Helen Young

First published in the United States in 1988 by Henry Holt and
Company, Inc., 115 West 18th Street, New York, New York 10011.
First published in Great Britain in 1986
by Dorling Kindersley Limited, London.

Library of Congress Catalog Card Number: 87-45841

ISBN 0-8050-2215-5 (An Owl Book: pbk.)

Henry Holt books are available at special discounts for bulk
purchases for sales promotions, premiums, fund-raising, or
educational use. Special editions or book excerpts can also be
created to specification.

For details contact:
Special Sales Director
Henry Holt and Company, Inc.
115 West 18th Street
New York, New York 10011

Second American Edition

Printed in Italy
1 3 5 7 9 10 8 6 4 2

Contents

Introduction

Why yet another book about sex? Sexual relationships and the difficulties surrounding them assume major importance in many people's lives. Yet it is only in the past 15 years that satisfactory short-term and direct-treatment procedures have been available, and it has taken this time to evaluate their active ingredients effectively and to put their relative merits in perspective. Since the spread of the AIDS virus there has also been a need for greater awareness about how our sex lives can affect our health, and what we can do to make sex safer.

Most people do not, in fact, have specific sexual problems, but have instead nagging difficulties or discrepancies with respect to their partners; for example, an inability to relax, a reluctance to engage in adequate foreplay or afterplay, the loss of sexual attraction to one another, or simply difficulty in keeping a relationship alive. And yet this book does not assume that every reader already has a sexual partner. Indeed, a whole section addresses single men, particularly those who have difficulty in finding a partner.

Sexual problems

This book deals with the rich and diverse pattern of human sexuality, but places special emphasis on its problems and their resolution. Whether you happen to be in your teens, the prime of life, or well advanced in years, are about to experience your first sexual encounter or have had such adventures many times before, you will find here practical advice. This is a book for everyone, irrespective of their age, race or sexual orientation.

Some how-to-do-it sex manuals offer ineffectual solutions to the reader's problems. Others, in hot pursuit of an illusory sexual excellence, bypass the question of emotional and functional difficulties altogether, as if they did not exist. What distinguishes this book from the vast majority is not just that it proposes effective remedies for sexual problems, but that it embodies a personalized approach. The problem charts, above all, probe behind common experiences to explore sexual difficulties on an individual level.

The questions in these charts are designed to pinpoint the particular characteristics of your problem, allowing you to examine your situation with some of the insight of the trained therapist. Accurate and early pinpointing is an important part of overcoming problems effectively and it cannot be overemphasized that rigorous self-assessment of this kind will minimize frustration and disappointment during the subsequent self-help programs.

The book is also different in structure. Lively features share space with highly practical questionnaires and the problem charts, both of which give easy access to precise and up-to-date information based on facts derived from clinical research of the past ten or so years.

This book is arranged systematically and it makes sense to use it similarly. The first part, YOUR SEXUAL PROFILE, will provide you with a picture of where you are right now in terms of sexual adjustment and competence. According to your scores for the question-naires, you will be guided to appropriate sections of the second part, PROBLEM CHARTS. These will enable you to diagnose your sexual difficulties and direct you to the third part, IMPROVING YOUR SEX LIFE, where there are appropriate exercise programs.

Enriching your sex life

The emphasis in this third part is on getting the most out of your sex life, regardless of whether or not you have a sexual problem. The aim is 'enrichment' rather than therapy, whether it be choosing a suitable position for intercourse, exploring your partner's erogenous zones, or learning to give yourself pleasure.

IMPROVING YOUR SEX LIFE also contains step-by-step instructions on how to resolve the specific sexual problems discussed in previous sections, using techniques that have been evaluated scientifically. Such problems usually persist where there are anxiety and guilt. This part of the book offers practical means of eliminating or relieving these negative emotional states.

Barriers to forming relationships

The fourth and fifth parts, THE MAN WITH A STEADY PARTNER and THE SINGLE MAN, are intended, respectively, for those who have a steady partner and those who do not. Traditionally, texts on sexual enrichment and therapy are aimed only at those already involved in a relationship, but we acknowledge that there are many who, for a variety of reasons, do not have a partner. Often, these reasons are related to sex. Experience has shown that once a sexual concern has been resolved, relationships are sought out more confidently. But we also appreciate that relationships themselves can conceal sexual difficulties.

The fourth part, being intended specifically for the man in a steady relationship, explores the major issues of compatibility and communication and helps the user gain a better understanding of female sexuality. At the same time, the potentially destructive problems of sexual boredom, infidelity and jealousy are confronted in depth. Finally, the full choice of contraceptive methods is covered, as are the lovemaking positions suitable in pregnancy.

The needs of the single man

The final part of the book, THE SINGLE MAN, contains a wealth of material relevant to both those who do not have a steady partner by choice and those who are single because they cannot integrate their social and sexual skills. Recommendations are given to men who have difficulty in finding or choosing a suitable partner, and to those who are embarking on a new sexual relationship.

The appendices suggest guidelines for safer sexual practices, give advice about conditions which may have an adverse effect on sexual functioning, and provide a brief survey of sexually transmitted diseases along with information on testing for AIDS. Finally, the Resource Guide suggests further reading and advises you on where you can obtain professional help for sexual problems.

If you simply read this book without doing any of the exercises, you will undoubtedly miss a great deal. Sexual happiness is everyone's right. By following the text in the way intended, and by putting into practice the relevant exercises, you will be helped toward this life-enriching goal, and will be sure to have many enjoyable experiences en route.

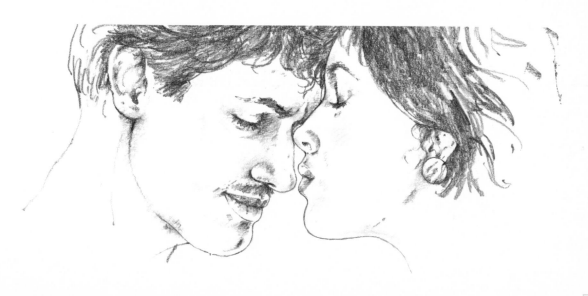

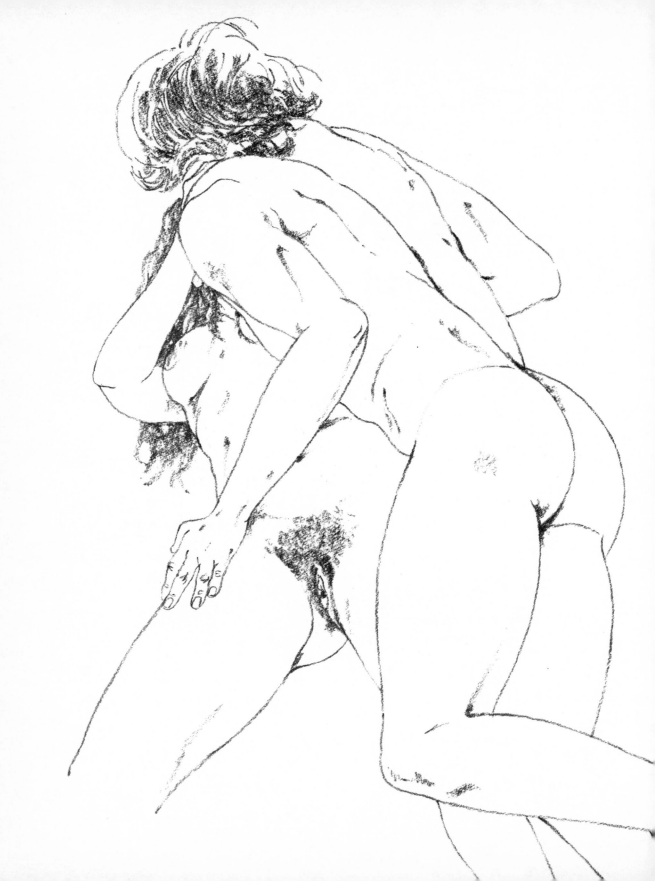

1

YOUR SEXUAL PROFILE

Your answers to the following questionnaires together form your sexual profile, a complete picture of the attitudes and behavior that shape your relationships and determine how much enjoyment you get and give in sex. By collating your scores for the questionnaires in the form of a chart, you can create your sexual profile. Instructions on how to do this are given on pp.20-1.

The answer to each question in the questionnaires on pp.10-18 carries a score. By checking your total score for a questionnaire against the **What you should do** box that follows it, you will obtain an assessment of where you stand in the particular area of your sex life under examination. The questionnaire on p.19, while contributing to an overall view of your sexual identity, is not rated in this way, and serves simply to establish your orientation.

A low or medium score for a questionnaire indicates that a particular aspect of your sexual experience is limiting your happiness. An appropriate course of action is suggested where necessary, the first step of which is usually to study other sections of the book. Often the situation is indeed remediable, and you can change almost any aspect of your sex life that is a problem. This book aims to help you do so.

SEXUAL KNOWLEDGE

How much do you know about sex and sexual physiology?

Indicate by a T or F in the box whether each of the statements below is
true or false. Compare your total score with the ratings following the questionnaire.

1 Circumcision makes the penis less sensitive. ☐

2 Masturbation is bad because it leads to a loss of interest in sex with a partner. ☐

3 A condom gives some protection against AIDS. ☐

4 Vasectomy (male sterilization) cannot usually be reversed. ☐

5 Vasectomy usually reduces a man's desire for sex. ☐

6 The withdrawal method is an effective form of contraception. ☐

7 Conception is most likely around the middle of your partner's menstrual cycle. ☐

8 Sexually transmitted diseases can be caught from a lavatory seat. ☐

9 Sexual abstinence is bad for you. ☐

10 A hairy chest is an indication of virility. ☐

11 If a man is potent (able to have intercourse) he is therefore fertile. ☐

12 A woman's urinary passage is separate from her vagina. ☐

13 Simultaneous orgasm is necessary for satisfactory sex. ☐

14 The clitoris is a small, sensitive organ situated within the inner vaginal lips. ☐

15 The outer vaginal lips are the same in every woman. ☐

16 Most women need clitoral stimulation as well as intercourse to reach orgasm. ☐

17 Sportsmen can conserve their strength by abstaining from sex before a big event. ☐

18 Sexual intercourse during menstruation does no physical harm to either partner. ☐

19 Women who have passed the menopause have little interest in sex. ☐

20 A 'frigid' woman cannot be aroused. ☐

For key to answers see p.19.

Give yourself a point for each correct answer.

WHAT YOU SHOULD DO

High rating (16-20) Now try the questionnaire TECHNIQUE, p.17, to make sure that your skill matches your grasp of theory.

Medium rating (9-15) Check wrong answers (see below) and try TECHNIQUE, p.17.

Low rating (0-8) Besides checking your wrong answers (see below) and trying the questionnaire TECHNIQUE, p.17, see the problem charts NEGATIVE FEELINGS, p.26, UNFULFILLED EXPECTATIONS, p.30, and MASTURBATION ANXIETY, p.34.

You will find full answers to the questions as follows:

Question **1** – p.77; **2** – p.34; **3** p.128; **4,5** – p.129; **6** – p.128; **7** – p.130; **8** – p.154; **9** – p.135; **10,11** – p.130; **12** – p.50; **13** – p.57; **14,15** – p.50; **16** – p.119; **17** – p.116; **18** – p.117; **19** – p.120; **20** – p.117.

SEX DRIVE

How strong is your appetite for sex?

For each of the following questions, circle the score to the right of your answer.
Compare your total score with the ratings following the questionnaire.

1 If you are under 55, do you have sex:

More than three times a week? _____ 2
Once or twice a week? _____ 1
Less than once a week? _____ 0

If you are 55 or over, do you have sex:

More than once a week? _____ 2
Once or twice every couple of weeks? _____ 1
Seldom or never? _____ 0

2 How often do you masturbate?

At least 4-6 times a week _____ 2
Once a week or less _____ 0
Two or three times a week _____ 1

3 Did you first have sexual intercourse:

Earlier than most of your friends? _____ 2
Around the time that most of your friends
    were starting to have sex? _____ 1
At a later age than most of your friends? _____ 0

4 Do you have genital stirrings when not consciously thinking of sex:

Once or twice a week? _____ 1
Most days? _____ 2
Seldom or never? _____ 0

5 Do you have erection problems?

Not very often _____ 1
Seldom or never _____ 2
Often _____ 0

6 Do you fantasize about sex (apart from when masturbating or making love):

Very often? _____ 2
Sometimes? _____ 1
Seldom or never? _____ 0

7 Do you think about sex:

Several times a day? _____ 2
Most days? _____ 1
Seldom or never? _____ 0

8 Have you been sexually involved with more than one person at a time:

Several times? _____ 2
Seldom? _____ 1
Never? _____ 0

9 Do erotic magazines:

Always excite you? _____ 2
Not turn you on at all? _____ 0
Sometimes excite you? _____ 1

10 Are your close relationships mainly:

Sexual? _____ 2
Tinged with a strong sexual element? _____ 1
Just friendly without sexual overtones? _____ 0

WHAT YOU SHOULD DO

High rating (16-20) You have a strong sex drive, which is fine if you have a partner who satisfies you.

Medium rating (9-15) Your sex drive should be no bar to sexual satisfaction. You can confirm this by doing the questionnaire ARE YOU SEXUALLY SATISFIED?, p.109.

Low rating (0-8) Consult the problem chart LACK OF INTEREST, p.24. In many cases a lack of sex drive presents no problems, but check if it is a symptom of illness. See SEX AND HEALTH, p.151.

PSYCHOLOGICAL WELL-BEING

Can you enjoy sex without anxiety or guilt?

For each question, circle the appropriate score. Compare your
total score with the ratings following the questionnaire.

	YES	NO		YES	NO
1 Do you feel sex is unimportant and has never played a large part in your life?	0	1	**6** Do you worry about catching AIDS, though you are not in a high risk group?	0	1
2 Are you a solitary person, unable or unwilling to get emotionally close to others?	0	1	**7** Are you usually confident of your ability to perform sexually?	1	0
3 Would you describe yourself as a jealous person?	0	1	**8** Are you completely sure about your preference for heterosexual relationships to homosexual ones, or vice versa?	1	0
4 Do you feel that unless you control yourself, sex might dominate your life?	0	1	**9** Do you often feel difficulty in living up to the masculine role expected of you?	0	1
5 Do you find sex messy? Are you repelled by the sight, odor, and feel of seminal or vaginal fluid, for example, or do you feel uneasy unless you can take a bath or shower right after intercourse?	0	1	**10** Does the idea of unusual sexual practices (involving violence or underage partners, for example) excite you more than the thought of conventional sex?	0	1

WHAT YOU SHOULD DO

High rating (8-10)

You are able to relax and respond naturally in a sexual situation. However, sexual functioning is very easily thrown off balance, so where you scored 0 on a question, consult the appropriate problem chart (see **Low rating**). This will help you to increase your sexual enjoyment even more.

Medium rating (5-7)

This suggests that fear or guilt about sex probably makes it hard for you to enjoy a sexual relationship fully. Consult the appropriate problem chart on the questions for which you scored 0 (see **Low rating**).

Low rating (0-4)

Your capacity for, and interest in, sex are needlessly limited. The problem charts listed below deal with factors which commonly influence psychological health and attitudes to sex. Consult them as follows on questions for which you scored 0:

Question 1– LACK OF INTEREST, p.24; **2** – LACK OF EMOTIONAL INVOLVEMENT, p.28; **3** – LOW SELF-ESTEEM, p.32; **4-7** – NEGATIVE FEELINGS, p.26; **8,9** – HETEROSEXUALITY/HOMOSEXUALITY CONFLICTS, p.42; **10** – UNUSUAL SEXUAL PRACTICES, p.45.

SATISFACTION

Are you satisfied with your sex life?

For each question, circle the appropriate score. Compare your total score with the ratings following the questionnaire.

	YES	NO		YES	NO
1 Are you getting as much sex as you would like?	1	0	**6** Is sex usually as good as you had imagined it would be?	1	0
2 Are you getting the kind of sex you like, so that you usually do the things you most enjoy?	1	0	**7** Is sex always or frequently disappointing?	0	1
3 Does your usual sexual partner still arouse you?	1	0	**8** Do you usually feel relaxed, happy, and comfortable after sex?	1	0
4 Do you believe that most people get more excitement from sex than you do?	0	1	**9** Do you feel that your partner usually enjoys sex as much as you do?	1	0
5 Do you normally anticipate sex with great pleasure?	1	0	**10** Is your usual partner too sexually demanding?	0	1

WHAT YOU SHOULD DO

High rating (8-10)
You seem happy with both the quality and quantity of your sex life. If you have a regular sexual partner, do the questionnaire ARE YOU SEXUALLY SATISFIED?, p.109, together. This will give a measure of your sexual compatibility and show you whether your partner's satisfaction equals yours.

Medium rating (5-7)
Ask yourself whether the main source of dissatisfaction is your relationship with a particular person or whether you perhaps have an unrealistic idea of how great sex ought to be. The questionnaires COMPATIBILITY, p.104, and ARE YOU SEXUALLY SATISFIED?, p.109, will be helpful in the former case. In the latter case, the problem chart UNFULFILLED EXPECTATIONS, p.30, will help you develop a more realistic view of sex.

Low rating (0-4)
Besides consulting the questionnaires and problem chart referred to above, it is especially important to complete the other questionnaires in the first part of the book. Further low ratings may enable you to identify causes of your low level of satisfaction.

SENSUALITY

How important is bodily contact to you in a loving relationship?

For each question, circle the appropriate score. Compare your
total score with the ratings following the questionnaire.

	YES	NO		YES	NO
1 Do you know the erogenous zones of your own body (those areas that particularly arouse you when they are touched)?	1	0	**6** Do you often hug or kiss a lover simply to show affection, or just when you feel like sex?	1	0
2 Do you feel self-conscious or uncomfortable when your partner touches or caresses you after your orgasm?	0	1	**7** Do you like to hold hands or link arms when walking with a lover?	1	0
3 Are you physically demonstrative with people you are fond of, regardless of their sex?	1	0	**8** Do you prefer to make love in the nude?	1	0
4 Do you think it unmasculine to be physically demonstrative?	0	1	**9** After sex, do you dislike caressing your partner?	0	1
5 If you cannot sleep or are depressed, does it help to be held or to hold someone?	1	0	**10** Do you enjoy sleeping with your partner, whether or not you have had sex?	1	0

WHAT YOU SHOULD DO

High rating (8-10)
Sensuality and physical closeness, both vital in making rewarding sexual relationships, come easily to you. EXPANDING YOUR SEXUAL REPERTOIRE, p.48, will help you make the most of this ability.

Medium rating (5-7)
This suggests that you have the capacity for enjoying physical closeness but have not developed it sufficiently. If your sex life is not as fulfilling as you believe it could be, turn to the problem chart UNFULFILLED EXPECTATIONS, p.30, which will give you advice on how to improve the situation.

Low rating (0-4)
Your lack of physical demonstrativeness probably reflects an emotional coolness which could seriously affect your capacity to make close relationships. The problem chart LACK OF EMOTIONAL INVOLVEMENT, p.28, will help you to develop a greater capacity for closeness.

COMMUNICATION

How well can you communicate – both verbally and non-verbally – with your sexual partner?

For each question, circle the appropriate score. Compare your
total score with the ratings following the questionnaire.

	YES	NO		YES	NO
1 Do you usually talk with a partner about her and your own likes and dislikes in lovemaking?	1	0	**6** Do you find it difficult to make up after a quarrel?	0	1
2 Have you ever told a partner about your sexual fantasies?	1	0	**7** Are you capable of telling your partner that you love her?	1	0
3 If a partner wants sex but you are not in the mood, can you indicate this without making her feel rejected?	1	0	**8** Would you be embarrassed to tell a new partner you prefer to use a condom to reduce the risk of AIDS?	0	1
4 If you have a temporary sexual difficulty – an inability to get an erection, for example – can you discuss it freely with your partner?	1	0	**9** If your partner is hurt or angry, do you often react by becoming angry yourself?	0	1
5 Are you reluctant to express anger or hurt because you fear that it might harm your relationship?	0	1	**10** Do you always discuss contraception with a new partner?	1	0

WHAT YOU SHOULD DO

High rating (8-10)
You obviously communicate well with your partner, but EXPANDING YOUR SEXUAL REPERTOIRE, p.48, may help you to make even more of this ability.

Medium rating (5-7)
You are slightly inhibited when it comes to communication with a partner. The problem chart NEGATIVE FEELINGS, p.26, examines some of the reasons for this and directs you to helpful features.

Low rating (0-4)
Because you lack the ability to express yourself, you are missing out on a vital element in successful sexual relationships. Turn to problem chart LACK OF EMOTIONAL INVOLVEMENT, p.28.

CONFIDENCE

How do you rate your sex appeal and ability as a lover?

For each question, circle the appropriate score. Compare your total score with the ratings following the questionnaire.

	YES	NO		YES	NO
1 Do you often avoid asking for a date because you are afraid that you will be turned down?	0	1	**6** Do you think it is more important to please your partner than to achieve satisfaction for yourself?	0	1
2 Do you feel that your penis is smaller than other men's?	0	1	**7** If your partner suggested that you change your sexual routine, would you be likely to take it as a criticism of your ability as a lover?	0	1
3 Are you uncomfortable about being naked in front of your partner?	0	1	**8** Are you frightened of being rejected if you suggest a change in your sexual routine?	0	1
4 Do you sometimes avoid intercourse because you doubt your competence?	0	1	**9** When things go wrong with your relationship, do you always, or most often, assume it is your fault?	0	1
5 Do you believe you are as good a lover as most other men?	1	0	**10** Do you seldom feel jealous?	1	0

WHAT YOU SHOULD DO

High rating (8-10)

You are obviously confident in your sexual relationships. Sometimes, though, too much self-confidence can make you rather unaware of others' feelings. If your relationships seldom last long, see the problem chart DIFFICULTY IN SUSTAINING RELATIONSHIPS, p.140, which may help you pinpoint the reasons for this.

Medium rating (5-7)

Your slight lack of self-confidence may make you shy and even cause you to seem unfriendly to others. If so, consult the problem chart LOW SELF-ESTEEM, p.32, which will direct you toward helpful features. If you feel that your diffidence limits your sexual experience, see the section on DIFFICULTY IN FORMING SEXUAL RELATIONSHIPS, p.138.

Low rating (0-4)

A poor self-image may be limiting your social as well as your sexual enjoyment. Begin by consulting the problem chart LOW SELF-ESTEEM, p.32. But if your problem is so severe that it prevents you forming relationships, you should read DIFFICULTY IN FINDING A PARTNER, p.136.

TECHNIQUE

How capable are you of arousing and satisfying a partner?

For each question, circle the appropriate score. Compare your total score with the ratings following the questionnaire.

	YES	NO		YES	NO
1 Are you able to delay your orgasm in order to prolong intercourse?	1	0	**6** Do you find leisurely foreplay a waste of time or frustrating?	0	1
2 Does it trouble you if your partner tries to initiate sex?	0	1	**7** After sex, do you always cuddle your partner affectionately?	1	0
3 Do you often find it difficult to achieve or sustain an erection?	0	1	**8** Do you genuinely like women and enjoy their company?	1	0
4 Have you varied your lovemaking technique over the last six months by, for example, trying a new position or simply having sex in a different place or at an unusual time?	1	0	**9** When you have an orgasm during intercourse and your partner does not, do you usually try to satisfy her by other means?	1	0
5 Do you always make sure a woman is fully aroused before you penetrate her?	1	0	**10** Do you normally take the trouble to create a romantic setting or mood as a prelude to sex?	1	0

WHAT YOU SHOULD DO

High rating (8-10)
You are obviously a competent lover. But love-making is a subtle skill. Therefore, if your scores for the questionnaires SENSUALITY, p.14, and COMMUNICATION, p.15, are considerably lower than your score here, you probably need to develop your ability to make your partner feel emotionally, as well as physically, fulfilled. Follow the advice given in the ratings guides to these questionnaires.

Medium rating (5-7)
You may well have inhibitions which affect your sexual skill. Consult the problem chart NEGATIVE FEELINGS, p.26. It may be, though, that your real problem is simply inexperience. The problem chart UNFULFILLED EXPECTATIONS, p.30, will direct you to helpful features.

Low rating (0-4)
Do not be discouraged by your low score. Sexual technique can be learned and it is never too late. It is also important to examine your feelings about sex (see NEGATIVE FEELINGS, p.26, and UNFUL-FILLED EXPECTATIONS, p.30). However, if it seems that your problems are predominantly a matter of technique rather than attitude, they are most likely dealt with in ERECTION PRO-BLEMS, p.36, and PREMATURE EJACULA-TION, p.38.

BROADMINDEDNESS

How tolerant of sexual freedom and experimentation are you?

For each question, circle the appropriate score. Compare your
total score with the ratings following the questionnaire.

	YES	NO		YES	NO
1 Do you prefer to make love with the light on?	1	0	**6** Do you enjoy oral sex?	1	0
2 Do you think a partner's infidelity is a good enough reason to end an otherwise happy relationship?	0	1	**7** Do sexually explicit movies, magazines, or books embarrass you?	0	1
3 Does anything other than the male-on-top position seem wrong to you?	0	1	**8** Have you tried anal sex?	1	0
4 Would you think less of a friend if you discovered he was homosexual?	0	1	**9** Have you tried group sex?	1	0
5 Have you ever used a mirror to watch yourself making love?	1	0	**10** Have you ever acted out any of your sexual fantasies with a partner?	1	0

WHAT YOU SHOULD DO

High rating (8-10)

You have a very tolerant attitude toward sexual self-expression. However, are you quite sure your interest in novelty does not suggest a degree of boredom with your present sex life? If your rating for the questionnaire SATISFACTION, p.13, is not equally high, turn to the problem chart UNFUL-FILLED EXPECTATIONS, p.30, which suggests possible reasons for dissatisfaction and features which will help you overcome it. If you answered "Yes" to questions eight or nine you might be a little more cautious in your approach to sex. Both of these are 'high risk' activities as far as AIDS is concerned. The use of a condom and spermicide can reduce the dangers, but the safest sexual relationships are those in which neither partner has any other sexual contacts. Resist pressure to be 'broadminded' if it involves doing anything you feel is dangerous or anything that simply does not appeal to you.

Medium rating (5-7)

You are probably reasonably happy with your cautious attitude toward sex. But if you find you have lost some of your enthusiasm, turn to the problem chart LACK OF INTEREST, p.24. Perhaps you have never found sex very exciting, in which case the problem chart UNFULFILLED EXPEC-TATIONS, p.30, will help you.

Low rating (0-4)

You are undoubtedly too cautious about sex, and perhaps even find it sinful or shameful. Such attitudes are almost certainly limiting your sexual happiness. The problem chart NEGATIVE FEELINGS, p.26, will direct you to features that will help you develop a more balanced outlook. See also the questionnaire PSYCHOLOGICAL WELL-BEING, p.12.

ORIENTATION

Are your sexual inclinations heterosexual, homosexual, or somewhere between the two?

Read through the statements and choose the one that most accurately describes you.
If you have no sexual experience, try to imagine what your inclinations might be.

	RATING		RATING
I am sexually aroused only by, and have sex only with, women.	A	I have sex with both men and women, but my sexual fantasies are more often about men.	E
I am sexually aroused by women, but have occasional fantasies of sex with men.	B	I prefer men and have little interest in women as sexual partners.	F
I prefer sex with women, but have occasional homosexual encounters that mean little to me.	C	I am sexually aroused only by, and have sex only with, men.	G
I am equally aroused by men and women and enjoy sex with both.	D		

WHAT YOU SHOULD DO

Your choice among the above statements gives you a rating on a scale of sexual orientation adapted from the one devised by the sexologist Alfred Kinsey. To check your rating, turn to p.160. The ratings are not value judgments; if you are comfortable with your orientation, you need do nothing about it. But if you find it hard to reconcile your sexual inclinations with other areas of your life, study the problem chart HETEROSEXUALITY/HOMOSEXUALITY CONFLICTS, p.42.

KEY TO SEXUAL KNOWLEDGE QUESTIONNAIRE (p.10)

TRUE: Questions 3, 4, 7, 12, 14, 16, 18

FALSE: Questions 1, 2, 5, 6, 8, 9, 10, 11, 13, 15, 17, 19, 20

THE SEXUAL PROFILE CHART

Using the blank chart on p.160 (or a photocopy), indicate your score for each of the questionnaires by marking the appropriate point on the rating scale. Join the points to create your sexual profile.

Your rating for sexual satisfaction is the touchstone of this exercise. What you will probably find is that alongside factors that contribute to your satisfaction there are others that are clearly limiting it.

Your scores for the four questionnaires on the right-hand side of the chart – **Psychological well-being**, **Confidence**, **Broadmindedness**, and **Sex drive** – reflect your fundamental attitudes to sex. High scores here indicate that you are sexually confident, while low scores suggest that you are perhaps inhibited in this area or have little interest in sex. (These factors are often linked, since a consistent lack of enthusiasm can conceal powerful inhibitions.) The questionnaires on the left-hand side of the graph – **Sensuality**, **Communication**, **Technique,** and **Sexual knowledge** – deal with those aspects of your sexual identity that are likely to affect your technique and your ability to be close to a partner.

Low scores in any part of your profile chart indicate problems, and advice is given in the ratings guides following the questionnaires. A serious imbalance in your scores is also a cause for concern. For example, it is possible to enjoy high confidence which conceals from you a poor grasp of sexual technique or an inability to understand another person's feelings. Similarly, your sexual knowledge may be extensive but you may lack confidence so that it is rarely, or never, put into practice.

It is possible for you to score low in one area without your being aware of the need – or simply the scope – for improvement in another. In this connection, it is particularly important to realize that while you may score low on the right-hand side and nevertheless feel sexually satisfied, your partner may remain unfulfilled. Accordingly, a lack of sexual confidence or a narrow-minded outlook may well underlie an inability to express warmth to your partner or may create difficulties in the practical aspects of lovemaking. Such problems will be reflected in low scores in the relevant areas on the left of the chart.

In a similar way you may be untroubled by a low score low on communication or on sensuality, since many men find it hard to talk about their feelings or to express physical (but not necessarily sexual) tenderness.

SAMPLE PROFILE CHARTS

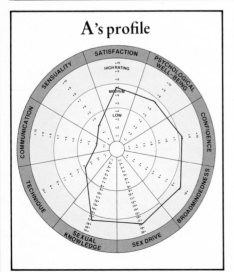

A's profile

A sees himself as very 'macho'. He has a strong sex drive, plenty of confidence, and is both experienced and knowledgeable. Yet his satisfaction rating is medium. He has never married and his relationships with women tend to be passionate but brief. Understandably, he has begun to wonder why they do not last.

There is a distinct imbalance in A's profile. While the right side betrays no obvious sexual hang-ups, the low ratings on the left indicate that, although he is by no means ignorant or a slow starter in matters of sex, he cannot easily communicate his feelings. In fact, it seldom occurs to A to show affection to his partner, or to acknowledge hers, except during sex.

A needs to learn to become more emotionally close to a partner. The problem chart LACK OF EMOTIONAL INVOLVEMENT, p.28, and the feature UNDERSTANDING A WOMAN'S FEELINGS, p.117, will help him understand that a sexual relationship is a two-way affair. By allowing himself to be more open with a woman and by appreciating her feelings, he will increase his pleasure and the chances of a stable relationship.

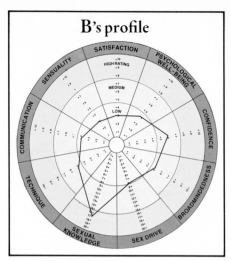

B's profile

B's satisfaction rating is low, and the uniformly poor ratings on the left side of his profile reinforce the suggestion that his relationship is very inadequate. The right side, however, shows low ratings for psychological well-being and broadmindedness, which together point to a problem in his feelings about sex.

In fact, B has strong homosexual leanings (indicated by an E rating on the Orientation questionnaire) which he finds it hard to acknowledge. He married partly to demonstrate his 'normality' and, sexually, the relationship has never been satisfactory.

The problem chart HETEROSEXUALITY/HOMOSEXUALITY CONFLICTS, p.42, and the feature COMING TO TERMS WITH HOMOSEXUALITY, p.97, will help B gauge the strength of his homosexual feelings and discover what kind of lifestyle he wants. His generally ambivalent attitude to sex will need to be resolved, however, if he is to make a success of any sexual relationship. The problem chart NEGATIVE FEELINGS, p.26, will help him to do this.

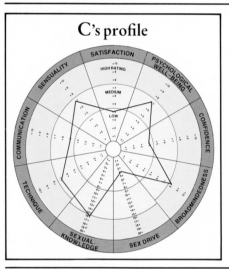

C's profile

C has an unexpectedly low satisfaction rating. The medium ratings on the left side of his profile suggest that he is a competent lover and able to make and sustain sexual relationships. But the right side shows a surprising lack of confidence and drive. C's relationship has deteriorated since, during a period of overwork and worry, he was several times unable to gain an erection. Each failure increased his anxiety about becoming impotent and eventually his fears became so intense that he avoided sex altogether. Because C found it hard to talk about the problem, his partner began to believe that he no longer loved or trusted her, and her own distress has driven a further wedge between them.

The problem chart ERECTION PROBLEMS, p.36 will reassure C that his temporary difficulty is unlikely to develop into a permanent problem unless he continues to worry about it. He would also do well to study LEARNING TO COMMUNICATE, p.114, which will help him overcome his inhibitions about speaking frankly about his feelings.

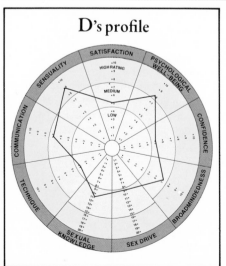

D's profile

D is in his teens and having his first sexual relationship. The right side of his profile points to a positive and enthusiastic attitude to sex. The absence of hang-ups, combined with high ratings for sensuality and communication, mean that he will probably find future sexual relationships easy. But, on the left, his relatively low ratings for knowledge and technique suggest that he experiences 'technical' difficulties when making love.

The fact is that D's eagerness and inexperience lead him to ejaculate prematurely. Understandably, this is affecting his self-confidence and explains why he does not find sex particularly satisfying at present.

Nevertheless, D's profile should reassure him that, sexually, he has good prospects and no reason to lack confidence. The problem chart PREMATURE EJACULATION, p.38, will confirm that his difficulty is one that will almost certainly disappear as his experience grows, whether the present relationship lasts or not. The chart also directs him to advice that will help him start dealing with the problem right away.

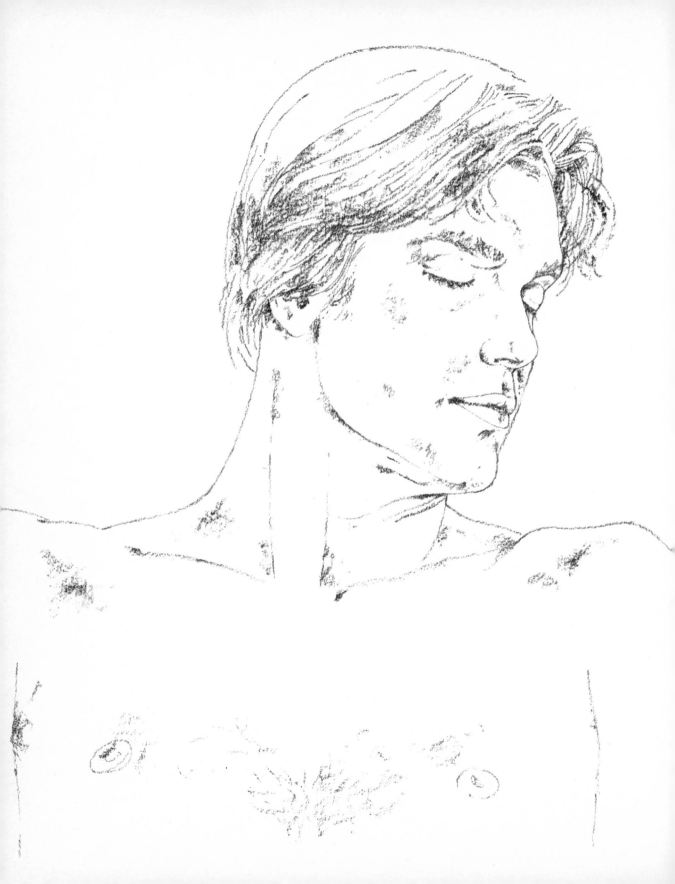

2

PROBLEM CHARTS

Each of the following self-diagnostic problem charts will help you track down the reasons for a particular sexual difficulty and offer you advice on resolving it. By means of a logically constructed network of questions to be answered either with a YES or a NO, the fourteen charts will lead you to conclusions based on authoritative research and expert opinion. Always begin at the first question and follow through to the correct endpoint for your special set of circumstances. The endpoint that you reach will either provide brief advice or, more often, refer you to other parts of the book where the problem is discussed in greater detail and self-help programs are given. Follow up cross-references in every case, so as not to miss further advice. In a few instances you may be advised to make use of a related problem chart or, occasionally, to seek professional help.

LACK OF INTEREST

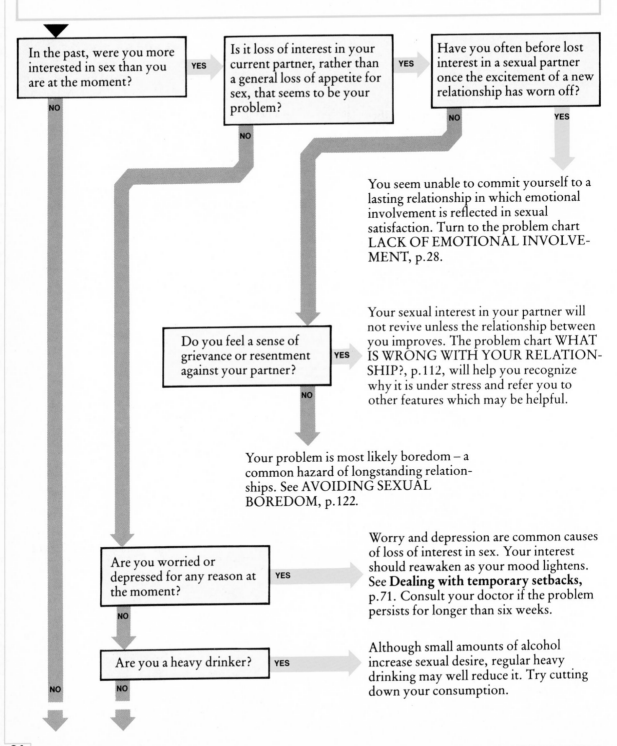

In the past, were you more interested in sex than you are at the moment?

YES →

Is it loss of interest in your current partner, rather than a general loss of appetite for sex, that seems to be your problem?

YES →

Have you often before lost interest in a sexual partner once the excitement of a new relationship has worn off?

YES

You seem unable to commit yourself to a lasting relationship in which emotional involvement is reflected in sexual satisfaction. Turn to the problem chart LACK OF EMOTIONAL INVOLVEMENT, p.28.

Do you feel a sense of grievance or resentment against your partner?

YES

Your sexual interest in your partner will not revive unless the relationship between you improves. The problem chart WHAT IS WRONG WITH YOUR RELATIONSHIP?, p.112, will help you recognize why it is under stress and refer you to other features which may be helpful.

Your problem is most likely boredom – a common hazard of longstanding relationships. See AVOIDING SEXUAL BOREDOM, p.122.

Are you worried or depressed for any reason at the moment?

YES

Worry and depression are common causes of loss of interest in sex. Your interest should reawaken as your mood lightens. See **Dealing with temporary setbacks,** p.71. Consult your doctor if the problem persists for longer than six weeks.

Are you a heavy drinker?

YES

Although small amounts of alcohol increase sexual desire, regular heavy drinking may well reduce it. Try cutting down your consumption.

NO **NO** **NO** **NO** **NO** **NO**

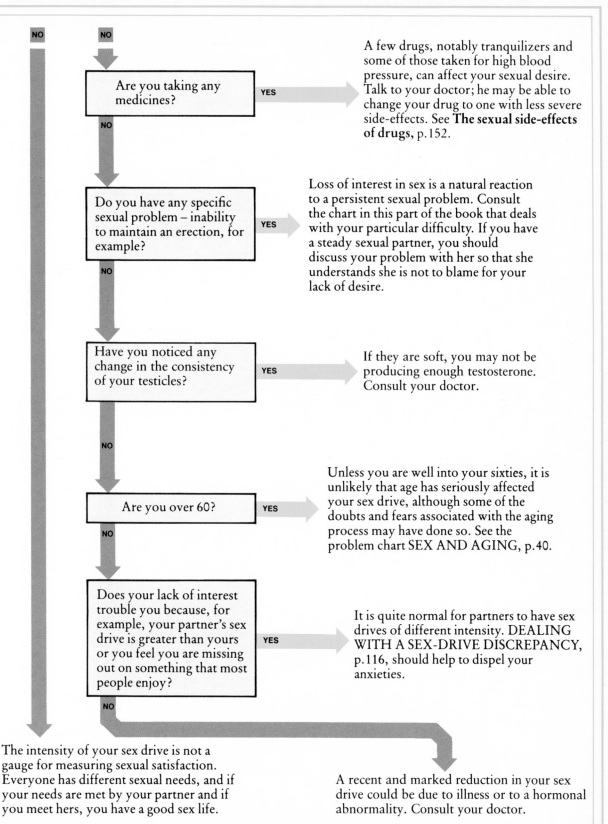

Are you taking any medicines?

YES → A few drugs, notably tranquilizers and some of those taken for high blood pressure, can affect your sexual desire. Talk to your doctor; he may be able to change your drug to one with less severe side-effects. See **The sexual side-effects of drugs**, p.152.

Do you have any specific sexual problem – inability to maintain an erection, for example?

YES → Loss of interest in sex is a natural reaction to a persistent sexual problem. Consult the chart in this part of the book that deals with your particular difficulty. If you have a steady sexual partner, you should discuss your problem with her so that she understands she is not to blame for your lack of desire.

Have you noticed any change in the consistency of your testicles?

YES → If they are soft, you may not be producing enough testosterone. Consult your doctor.

Are you over 60?

YES → Unless you are well into your sixties, it is unlikely that age has seriously affected your sex drive, although some of the doubts and fears associated with the aging process may have done so. See the problem chart SEX AND AGING, p.40.

Does your lack of interest trouble you because, for example, your partner's sex drive is greater than yours or you feel you are missing out on something that most people enjoy?

YES → It is quite normal for partners to have sex drives of different intensity. DEALING WITH A SEX-DRIVE DISCREPANCY, p.116, should help to dispel your anxieties.

The intensity of your sex drive is not a gauge for measuring sexual satisfaction. Everyone has different sexual needs, and if your needs are met by your partner and if you meet hers, you have a good sex life.

A recent and marked reduction in your sex drive could be due to illness or to a hormonal abnormality. Consult your doctor.

MEN ♂ 2 PROBLEM CHARTS

NEGATIVE FEELINGS

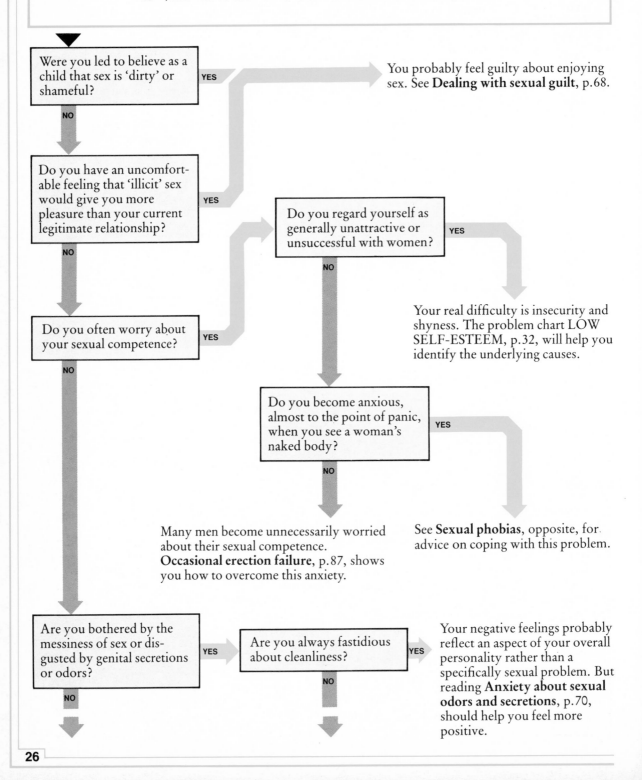

Were you led to believe as a child that sex is 'dirty' or shameful?

YES → You probably feel guilty about enjoying sex. See **Dealing with sexual guilt**, p.68.

NO ↓

Do you have an uncomfortable feeling that 'illicit' sex would give you more pleasure than your current legitimate relationship?

YES →

NO ↓

Do you regard yourself as generally unattractive or unsuccessful with women?

YES → Your real difficulty is insecurity and shyness. The problem chart LOW SELF-ESTEEM, p.32, will help you identify the underlying causes.

NO ↓

Do you often worry about your sexual competence?

YES →

NO ↓

Do you become anxious, almost to the point of panic, when you see a woman's naked body?

YES → See **Sexual phobias**, opposite, for advice on coping with this problem.

NO ↓

Many men become unnecessarily worried about their sexual competence. **Occasional erection failure**, p.87, shows you how to overcome this anxiety.

Are you bothered by the messiness of sex or disgusted by genital secretions or odors?

YES → Are you always fastidious about cleanliness?

YES → Your negative feelings probably reflect an aspect of your overall personality rather than a specifically sexual problem. But reading **Anxiety about sexual odors and secretions**, p.70, should help you feel more positive.

NO ↓ (Are you bothered by the messiness...)

NO ↓ (Are you always fastidious...)

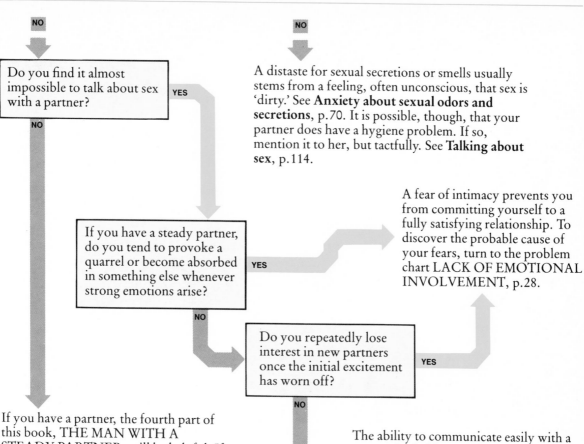

NO

Do you find it almost impossible to talk about sex with a partner?

YES

A distaste for sexual secretions or smells usually stems from a feeling, often unconscious, that sex is 'dirty.' See **Anxiety about sexual odors and secretions**, p.70. It is possible, though, that your partner does have a hygiene problem. If so, mention it to her, but tactfully. See **Talking about sex**, p.114.

NO

NO

If you have a steady partner, do you tend to provoke a quarrel or become absorbed in something else whenever strong emotions arise?

YES

A fear of intimacy prevents you from committing yourself to a fully satisfying relationship. To discover the probable cause of your fears, turn to the problem chart LACK OF EMOTIONAL INVOLVEMENT, p.28.

NO

Do you repeatedly lose interest in new partners once the initial excitement has worn off?

YES

NO

If you have a partner, the fourth part of this book, THE MAN WITH A STEADY PARTNER, will be helpful. If you do not have a partner, turn to the fifth part, THE SINGLE MAN.

The ability to communicate easily with a partner is vital for sustaining a close sexual relationship. See LEARNING TO COMMUNICATE, p.114.

SEXUAL PHOBIAS

A few men suffer anxiety so intense that it amounts to a phobia about part of the female body – usually the breasts or genitals – or about vaginal secretions. These feelings are nearly always part of a general view of sex as unclean or shameful, but this kind of phobia may indicate a general obsession with cleanliness.

However, genital phobia that arises from guilt or anxiety about sex can be overcome by a technique known as desensitization. This involves exposing yourself gradually to whatever it is that makes you feel uncomfortable, usually through visual images or your own fantasy. When your anxiety level has decreased you can start to face what you fear in reality.

Start by glancing through sexually explicit magazines. Then look at the pictures in more detail, gradually focusing more and more on the breasts and genitals but stopping to relax whenever your tension rises unbearably. Eventually (though it may take some weeks) you should be able to look at these and similar pictures without feeling uncomfortable and they may even start to make you feel sexually aroused. When you have reached this point, it will help your progress if you can masturbate, using the pictures as a stimulus to fantasy.

Likewise, take sex with a partner by stages, first caressing her clothed body, then, with her cooperation, doing the **Sensate-focusing exercises**, p.79. Remember that you have to push yourself a little to make your anxiety dissolve, but allow yourself to stop when you want to.

LACK OF EMOTIONAL INVOLVEMENT

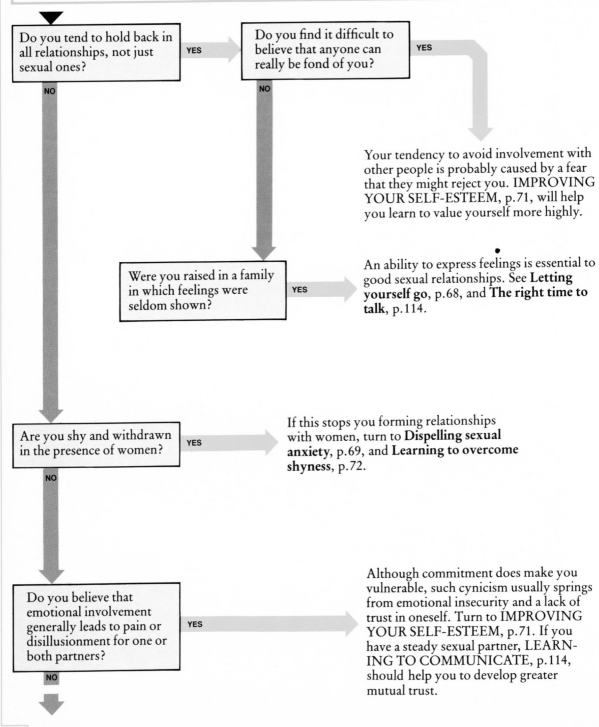

Do you tend to hold back in all relationships, not just sexual ones? — **YES** →

Do you find it difficult to believe that anyone can really be fond of you? — **YES** →

Your tendency to avoid involvement with other people is probably caused by a fear that they might reject you. IMPROVING YOUR SELF-ESTEEM, p.71, will help you learn to value yourself more highly.

NO ↓

Were you raised in a family in which feelings were seldom shown? — **YES** →

An ability to express feelings is essential to good sexual relationships. See **Letting yourself go**, p.68, and **The right time to talk**, p.114.

NO ↓

Are you shy and withdrawn in the presence of women? — **YES** →

If this stops you forming relationships with women, turn to **Dispelling sexual anxiety**, p.69, and **Learning to overcome shyness**, p.72.

NO ↓

Do you believe that emotional involvement generally leads to pain or disillusionment for one or both partners? — **YES** →

Although commitment does make you vulnerable, such cynicism usually springs from emotional insecurity and a lack of trust in oneself. Turn to IMPROVING YOUR SELF-ESTEEM, p.71. If you have a steady sexual partner, LEARN-ING TO COMMUNICATE, p.114, should help you to develop greater mutual trust.

NO ↓

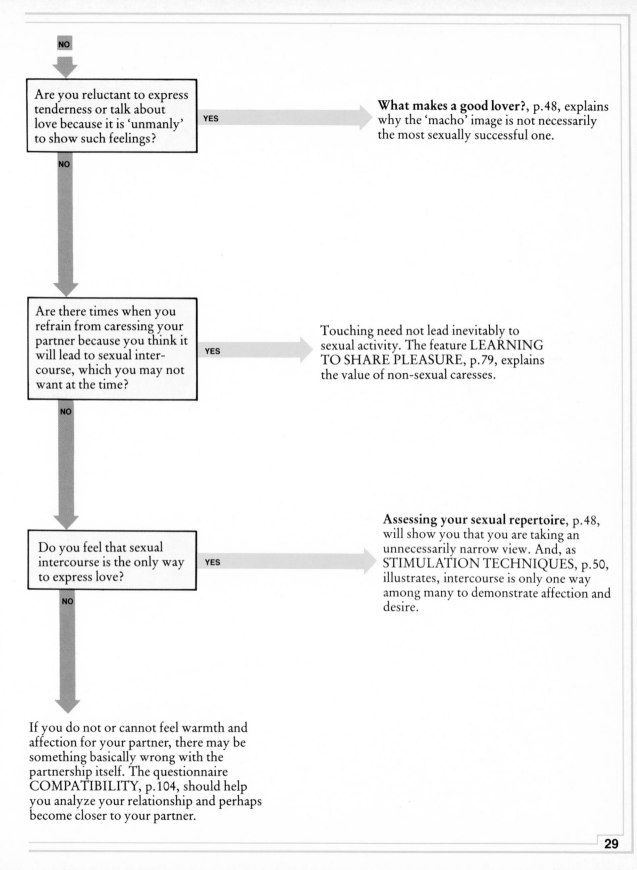

Are you reluctant to express tenderness or talk about love because it is 'unmanly' to show such feelings?

YES

What makes a good lover?, p.48, explains why the 'macho' image is not necessarily the most sexually successful one.

NO

Are there times when you refrain from caressing your partner because you think it will lead to sexual inter-course, which you may not want at the time?

YES

Touching need not lead inevitably to sexual activity. The feature LEARNING TO SHARE PLEASURE, p.79, explains the value of non-sexual caresses.

NO

Do you feel that sexual intercourse is the only way to express love?

YES

Assessing your sexual repertoire, p.48, will show you that you are taking an unnecessarily narrow view. And, as STIMULATION TECHNIQUES, p.50, illustrates, intercourse is only one way among many to demonstrate affection and desire.

NO

If you do not or cannot feel warmth and affection for your partner, there may be something basically wrong with the partnership itself. The questionnaire COMPATIBILITY, p.104, should help you analyze your relationship and perhaps become closer to your partner.

UNFULFILLED EXPECTATIONS

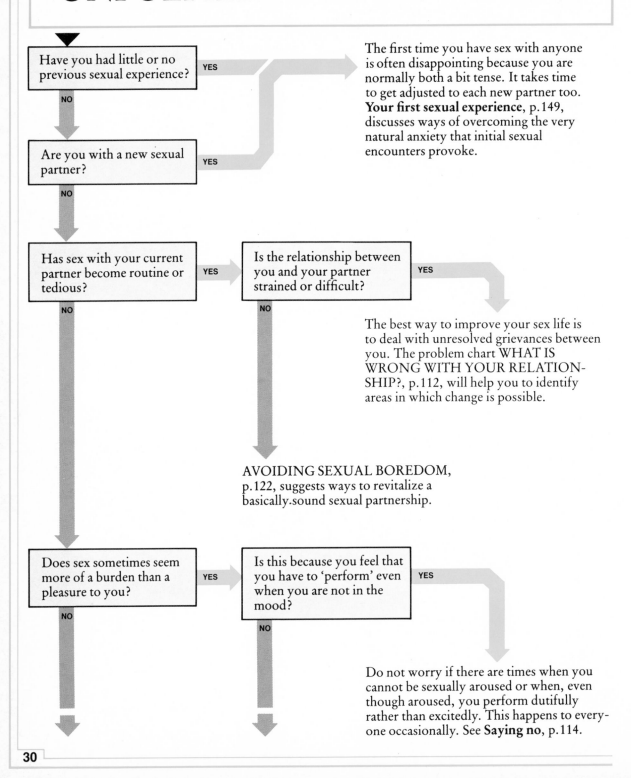

Have you had little or no previous sexual experience?

YES →

The first time you have sex with anyone is often disappointing because you are normally both a bit tense. It takes time to get adjusted to each new partner too. **Your first sexual experience**, p.149, discusses ways of overcoming the very natural anxiety that initial sexual encounters provoke.

NO

Are you with a new sexual partner?

YES →

NO

Has sex with your current partner become routine or tedious?

YES →

Is the relationship between you and your partner strained or difficult?

YES →

NO

The best way to improve your sex life is to deal with unresolved grievances between you. The problem chart WHAT IS WRONG WITH YOUR RELATION-SHIP?, p.112, will help you to identify areas in which change is possible.

NO

AVOIDING SEXUAL BOREDOM, p.122, suggests ways to revitalize a basically.sound sexual partnership.

Does sex sometimes seem more of a burden than a pleasure to you?

YES →

Is this because you feel that you have to 'perform' even when you are not in the mood?

YES →

NO

NO

Do not worry if there are times when you cannot be sexually aroused or when, even though aroused, you perform dutifully rather than excitedly. This happens to every-one occasionally. See **Saying no**, p.114.

Does sex frequently seem like a long hard struggle for orgasm?

YES

Take a lighter, more leisurely approach. If you have trouble achieving orgasm, enjoy physical contact for its own sake; your partner is unlikely to mind as long as you yourself have a relaxed and happy attitude. The problem chart RETARDED EJACULATION, p.39, should help you to discover why you have this trouble and to cope with it.

NO

An impression that sex is burdensome is often the result of not really getting the kind of sex you like. See **Assessing your sexual repertoire**, p.48.

Is there a lack of emotional closeness and satisfaction in your sexual relationships?

YES

Turn to the problem chart LACK OF EMOTIONAL INVOLVEMENT, p.28.

NO

Do you constantly change partners, hoping for more excitement, but feel let down after most sexual encounters?

YES

Good sex and good relationships take time to build. The problem chart WHY ARE YOU SINGLE?, p.134, will show you why you are unwilling to commit yourself fully to one person.

NO

Many men suspect that they are somehow missing out on the 'ultimate' sexual experience. However, the sensations of sex, as opposed to the emotions, are limited, and you perhaps have not yet accepted this fact. Even so, you might profit from experimenting with new sexual techniques. A rich variety of possibilities is discussed in EXPANDING YOUR SEXUAL REPERTOIRE, p.48.

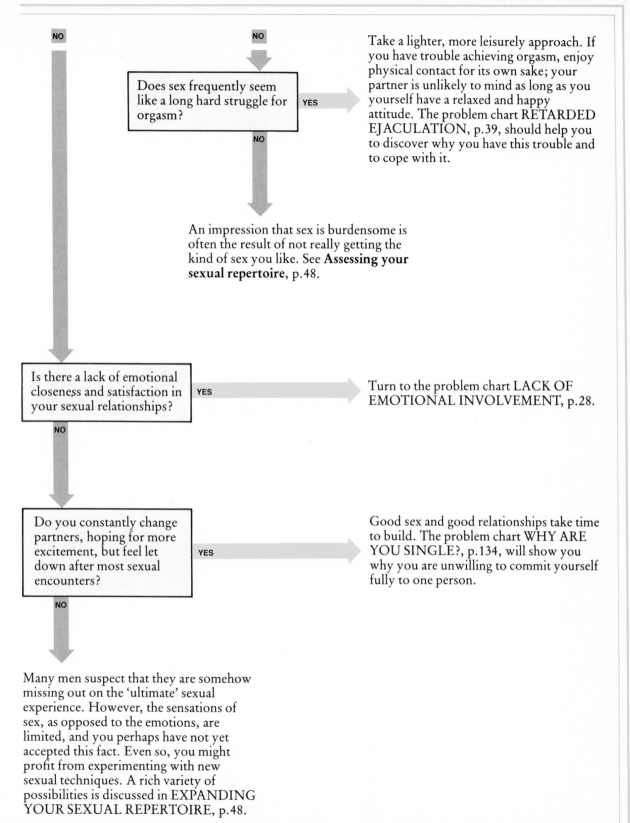

LOW SELF-ESTEEM

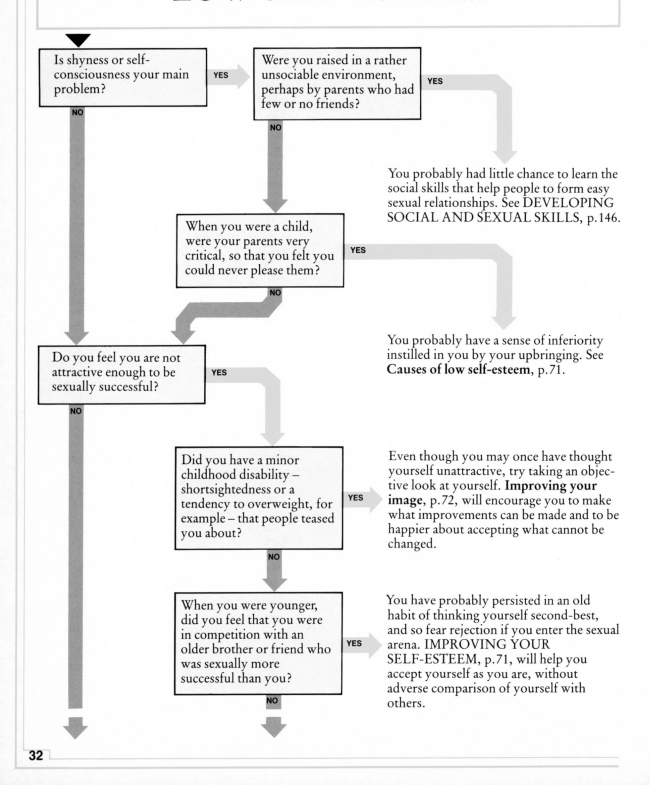

Is shyness or self-consciousness your main problem?

YES →

Were you raised in a rather unsociable environment, perhaps by parents who had few or no friends?

YES →

You probably had little chance to learn the social skills that help people to form easy sexual relationships. See DEVELOPING SOCIAL AND SEXUAL SKILLS, p.146.

NO ↓

When you were a child, were your parents very critical, so that you felt you could never please them?

YES →

You probably have a sense of inferiority instilled in you by your upbringing. See **Causes of low self-esteem**, p.71.

NO ↓

Do you feel you are not attractive enough to be sexually successful?

YES →

Did you have a minor childhood disability – shortsightedness or a tendency to overweight, for example – that people teased you about?

YES →

Even though you may once have thought yourself unattractive, try taking an objective look at yourself. **Improving your image**, p.72, will encourage you to make what improvements can be made and to be happier about accepting what cannot be changed.

NO ↓

When you were younger, did you feel that you were in competition with an older brother or friend who was sexually more successful than you?

YES →

You have probably persisted in an old habit of thinking yourself second-best, and so fear rejection if you enter the sexual arena. IMPROVING YOUR SELF-ESTEEM, p.71, will help you accept yourself as you are, without adverse comparison of yourself with others.

NO ↓

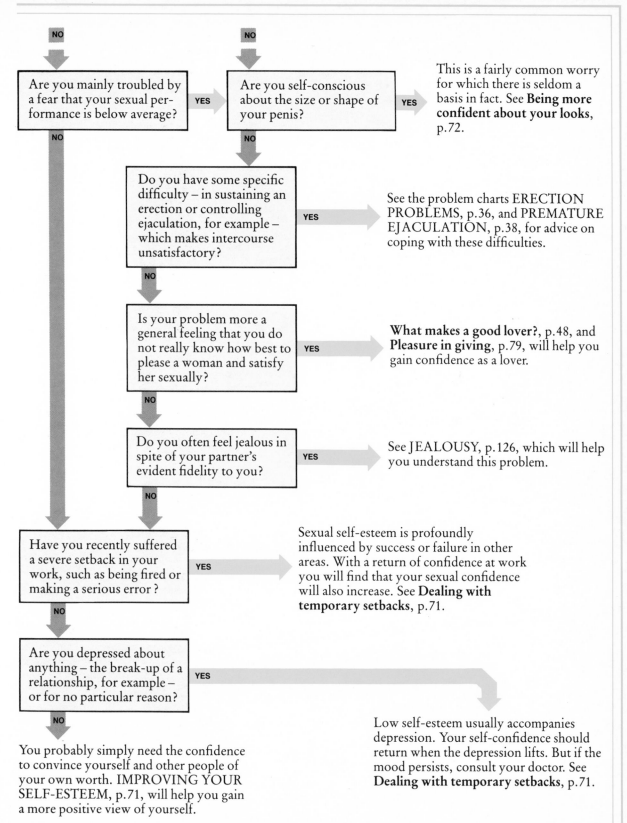

NO

Are you mainly troubled by a fear that your sexual performance is below average?

YES

NO

Are you self-conscious about the size or shape of your penis?

YES

This is a fairly common worry for which there is seldom a basis in fact. See **Being more confident about your looks,** p.72.

NO

Do you have some specific difficulty – in sustaining an erection or controlling ejaculation, for example – which makes intercourse unsatisfactory?

YES

See the problem charts ERECTION PROBLEMS, p.36, and PREMATURE EJACULATION, p.38, for advice on coping with these difficulties.

NO

Is your problem more a general feeling that you do not really know how best to please a woman and satisfy her sexually?

YES

What makes a good lover?, p.48, and **Pleasure in giving**, p.79, will help you gain confidence as a lover.

NO

Do you often feel jealous in spite of your partner's evident fidelity to you?

YES

See JEALOUSY, p.126, which will help you understand this problem.

NO

Have you recently suffered a severe setback in your work, such as being fired or making a serious error ?

YES

Sexual self-esteem is profoundly influenced by success or failure in other areas. With a return of confidence at work you will find that your sexual confidence will also increase. See **Dealing with temporary setbacks**, p.71.

NO

Are you depressed about anything – the break-up of a relationship, for example – or for no particular reason?

YES

NO

You probably simply need the confidence to convince yourself and other people of your own worth. IMPROVING YOUR SELF-ESTEEM, p.71, will help you gain a more positive view of yourself.

Low self-esteem usually accompanies depression. Your self-confidence should return when the depression lifts. But if the mood persists, consult your doctor. See **Dealing with temporary setbacks**, p.71.

MASTURBATION ANXIETY

Do you believe that masturbation causes physical or mental harm? — **YES** → None of the old notions about the damaging effects of masturbation is true. No matter how much you masturbate it will do you no harm. See GIVING YOURSELF PLEASURE, p.77.

NO ↓

Even though you know it is not harmful, do you feel guilty about masturbating? — **YES** → Many men feel uncomfortable about masturbating, while a few are reluctant to do it at all. Guilt can make you want to get it over quickly, and this is an attitude that may also make you overhasty in your approach to sex with a partner. OVERCOMING INHIBITIONS, p.68, will help you to review your attitude toward masturbation.

NO ↓

Do you experience pain when you masturbate? — **YES** → There are some physical conditions that make erection painful during any kind of sexual activity. Consult your doctor.

NO ↓

Do you impose limits on the amount that you masturbate? — **YES** → This is probably because you cannot escape feeling guilty about it. Frequent masturbation need only worry you if you find you are doing it much more than usual because you feel tense all the time. Such tension may be a symptom of anxiety and is something you should discuss with your doctor.

NO ↓

Do you believe that masturbation is justified only if you have no opportunity for sex with a partner? — **YES** → There is no need to regard masturbation as a substitute for 'real' sex, or to fear that it will lead to a loss of interest in it. At times it may simply be more convenient or suit your mood better than sex with a partner.

NO ↓

Nearly all men masturbate at least occasionally. Masturbation is most frequent during adolescence and among men without steady partners, but men in steady relationships also do it.

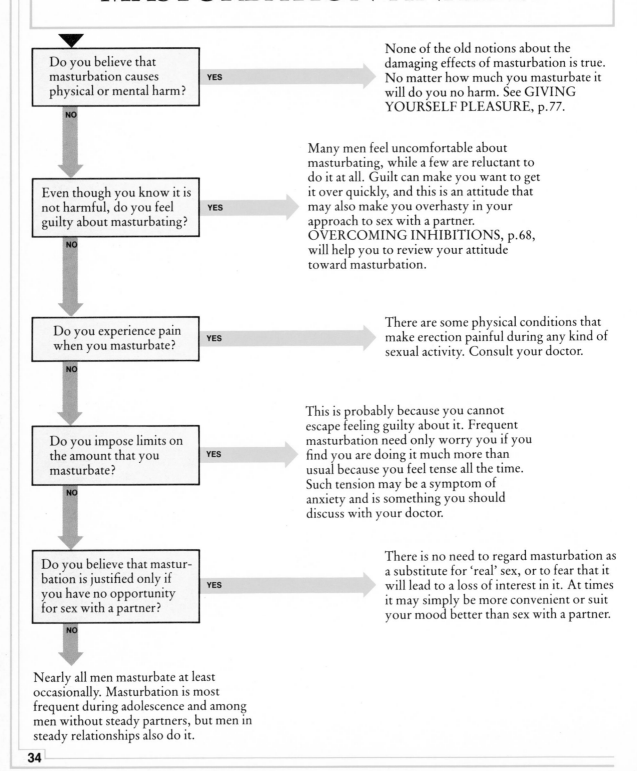

PAINFUL INTERCOURSE

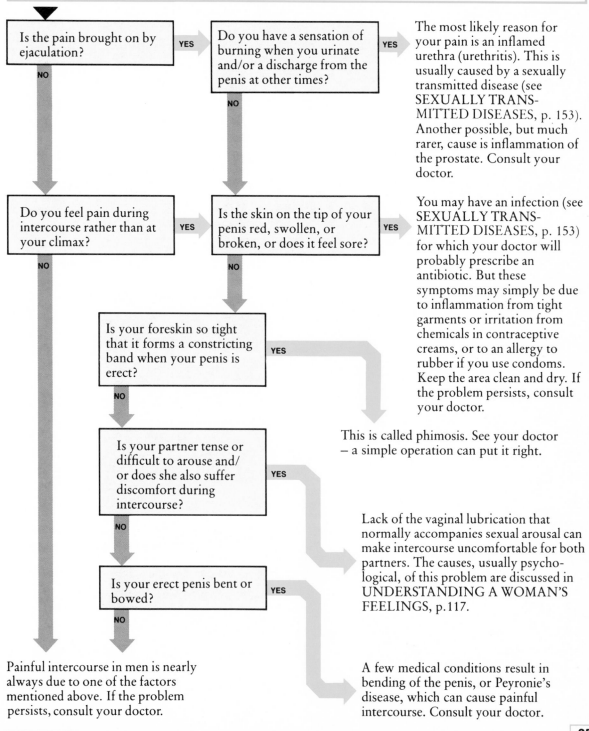

Is the pain brought on by ejaculation?

YES → Do you have a sensation of burning when you urinate and/or a discharge from the penis at other times?

YES → The most likely reason for your pain is an inflamed urethra (urethritis). This is usually caused by a sexually transmitted disease (see SEXUALLY TRANS-MITTED DISEASES, p. 153). Another possible, but much rarer, cause is inflammation of the prostate. Consult your doctor.

NO ↓

Do you feel pain during intercourse rather than at your climax?

YES → Is the skin on the tip of your penis red, swollen, or broken, or does it feel sore?

YES → You may have an infection (see SEXUALLY TRANS-MITTED DISEASES, p. 153) for which your doctor will probably prescribe an antibiotic. But these symptoms may simply be due to inflammation from tight garments or irritation from chemicals in contraceptive creams, or to an allergy to rubber if you use condoms. Keep the area clean and dry. If the problem persists, consult your doctor.

NO ↓

Is your foreskin so tight that it forms a constricting band when your penis is erect?

YES →

This is called phimosis. See your doctor – a simple operation can put it right.

NO ↓

Is your partner tense or difficult to arouse and/or does she also suffer discomfort during intercourse?

YES →

Lack of the vaginal lubrication that normally accompanies sexual arousal can make intercourse uncomfortable for both partners. The causes, usually psycho-logical, of this problem are discussed in UNDERSTANDING A WOMAN'S FEELINGS, p.117.

NO ↓

Is your erect penis bent or bowed?

YES →

NO ↓

Painful intercourse in men is nearly always due to one of the factors mentioned above. If the problem persists, consult your doctor.

A few medical conditions result in bending of the penis, or Peyronie's disease, which can cause painful intercourse. Consult your doctor.

ERECTION PROBLEMS

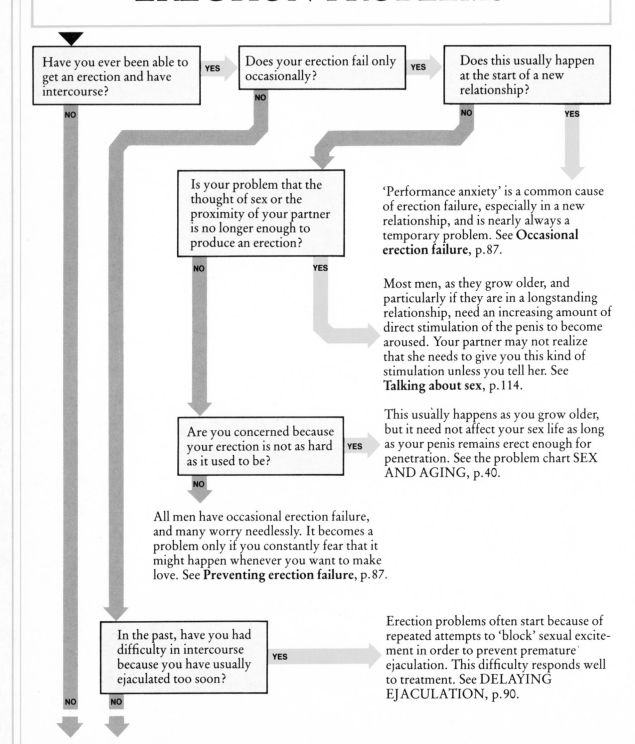

Have you ever been able to get an erection and have intercourse?

YES — Does your erection fail only occasionally?

YES — Does this usually happen at the start of a new relationship?

Is your problem that the thought of sex or the proximity of your partner is no longer enough to produce an erection?

'Performance anxiety' is a common cause of erection failure, especially in a new relationship, and is nearly always a temporary problem. See **Occasional erection failure**, p.87.

Most men, as they grow older, and particularly if they are in a longstanding relationship, need an increasing amount of direct stimulation of the penis to become aroused. Your partner may not realize that she needs to give you this kind of stimulation unless you tell her. See **Talking about sex**, p.114.

Are you concerned because your erection is not as hard as it used to be?

YES — This usually happens as you grow older, but it need not affect your sex life as long as your penis remains erect enough for penetration. See the problem chart SEX AND AGING, p.40.

All men have occasional erection failure, and many worry needlessly. It becomes a problem only if you constantly fear that it might happen whenever you want to make love. See **Preventing erection failure**, p.87.

In the past, have you had difficulty in intercourse because you have usually ejaculated too soon?

YES — Erection problems often start because of repeated attempts to 'block' sexual excitement in order to prevent premature ejaculation. This difficulty responds well to treatment. See DELAYING EJACULATION, p.90.

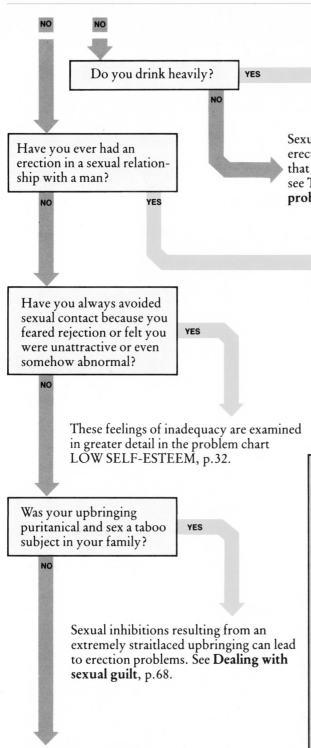

NO   NO

Do you drink heavily?   YES → Alcohol may affect your ability to achieve an erection and continual heavy drinking may cause permanent erection problems. See SEX AND HEALTH, p.151.

NO

Have you ever had an erection in a sexual relationship with a man? → Sexual anxiety is the root cause of most erection difficulties. If it happens so often that it is severely affecting your sex life, see **Treatment program for erection problems**, p.88.

NO   YES

If you have erection problems only with women, you obviously prefer male partners, whether or not you admit it to yourself. Consult the questionnaire ORIENTATION, p.19, which will help you decide the extent of your homosexuality. The problem chart HETEROSEXUALITY/HOMOSEXUALITY CONFLICTS, p.42, explores the difficulties you may have in accepting your homosexuality. See also COMING TO TERMS WITH HOMOSEXUALITY, p.97.

Have you always avoided sexual contact because you feared rejection or felt you were unattractive or even somehow abnormal?   YES

NO

These feelings of inadequacy are examined in greater detail in the problem chart LOW SELF-ESTEEM, p.32.

Was your upbringing puritanical and sex a taboo subject in your family?   YES

NO

Sexual inhibitions resulting from an extremely straitlaced upbringing can lead to erection problems. See **Dealing with sexual guilt**, p.68.

Erection failure is sometimes due to a hormonal or physical condition. Your doctor can arrange for tests to determine whether this is the cause of your problem.

OTHER CAUSES OF ERECTION PROBLEMS

Erection problems are not always 'in the mind'. Often they are caused by medical conditions, surgical operations, or drugs. See SEX AND HEALTH, p.151.

Mechanical devices such as the vacuum condom or the Blakoe ring are sometimes helpful. A more effective and increasingly widely used treatment is an injection, just before intercourse, of a drug which relaxes the smooth muscle of the arteries to the penis, increasing the blood flow. This method produces a good erection, but should not be used more than once a week.

When all other treatments fail, a special penile implant may be the answer. A semi-rigid rod is inserted, producing a penis stiff enough for intercourse, but not permanently and entirely erect. When not 'in use' it can be bent downwards so that it hangs normally.

PREMATURE EJACULATION

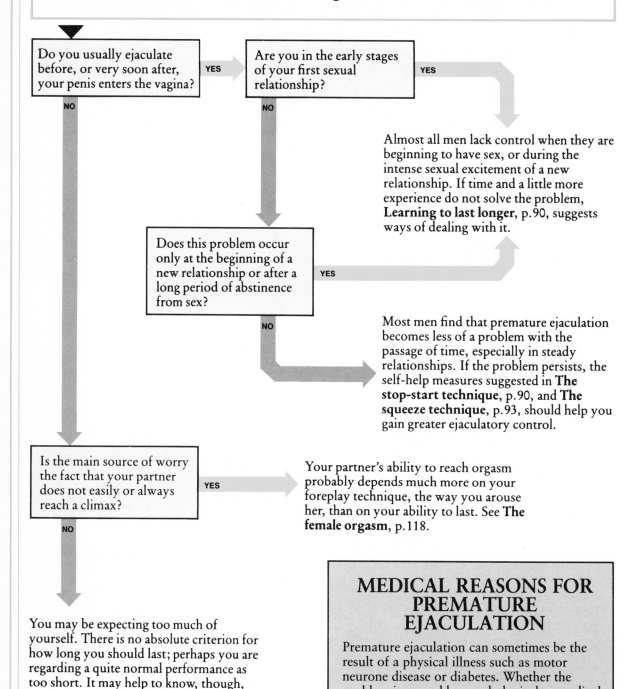

Do you usually ejaculate before, or very soon after, your penis enters the vagina?

YES →

Are you in the early stages of your first sexual relationship?

YES →

Almost all men lack control when they are beginning to have sex, or during the intense sexual excitement of a new relationship. If time and a little more experience do not solve the problem, **Learning to last longer**, p.90, suggests ways of dealing with it.

NO ↓

NO ↓

Does this problem occur only at the beginning of a new relationship or after a long period of abstinence from sex?

YES →

Most men find that premature ejaculation becomes less of a problem with the passage of time, especially in steady relationships. If the problem persists, the self-help measures suggested in **The stop-start technique**, p.90, and **The squeeze technique**, p.93, should help you gain greater ejaculatory control.

NO ↓

Is the main source of worry the fact that your partner does not easily or always reach a climax?

YES →

Your partner's ability to reach orgasm probably depends much more on your foreplay technique, the way you arouse her, than on your ability to last. See **The female orgasm**, p.118.

NO ↓

You may be expecting too much of yourself. There is no absolute criterion for how long you should last; perhaps you are regarding a quite normal performance as too short. It may help to know, though, that many men take longer to reach orgasm with their partner on top. See SEXUAL POSITIONS, p.55.

MEDICAL REASONS FOR PREMATURE EJACULATION

Premature ejaculation can sometimes be the result of a physical illness such as motor neurone disease or diabetes. Whether the problem is caused by psychological or medical factors, drug treatment can often help to bring it under control.

RETARDED EJACULATION

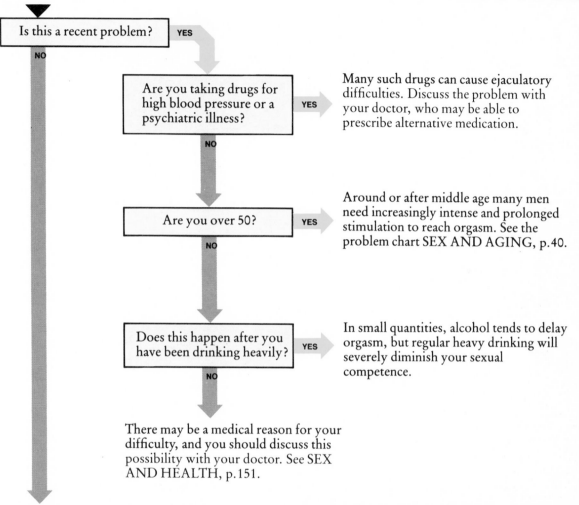

Is this a recent problem? — NO / YES

YES → Are you taking drugs for high blood pressure or a psychiatric illness?

YES → Many such drugs can cause ejaculatory difficulties. Discuss the problem with your doctor, who may be able to prescribe alternative medication.

NO ↓

Are you over 50?

YES → Around or after middle age many men need increasingly intense and prolonged stimulation to reach orgasm. See the problem chart SEX AND AGING, p.40.

NO ↓

Does this happen after you have been drinking heavily?

YES → In small quantities, alcohol tends to delay orgasm, but regular heavy drinking will severely diminish your sexual competence.

NO ↓

There may be a medical reason for your difficulty, and you should discuss this possibility with your doctor. See SEX AND HEALTH, p.151.

Your problem most likely stems from an inability to relax sexually. This tension often results from a sense of guilt or anxiety with its roots in childhood. See **Dealing with sexual guilt**, p.68. SPEEDING EJACULATION, p.95, suggests self-help measures for the physical aspects of the problem. It could be, however, that hostility to your partner, or to women in general, underlies your difficulty. See OVERCOMING THE FEAR OF INTIMACY, p.70, and DIFFICULTY IN SUSTAINING RELATIONSHIPS, p.140.

PROSTATECTOMY

Sometimes a man may be worried by an apparent absence of ejaculation after having a prostatectomy (surgical removal of the prostate gland). Without the prostate, seminal fluid may flow backward into the bladder instead of being ejaculated normally. When this, which is known as retrograde ejaculation, happens, the urine will look cloudy, but the backward flow is not harmful and the ability to experience orgasm is not affected.

SEX AND AGING

Do you believe that there is a medical reason why you cannot, or ought not to, engage in sexual activity at your age?

YES → Some physical conditions force older men to limit their sexual activity, but problems can nearly always be resolved without total abstinence. See SEX AND HEALTH, p.151.

NO ↓

Are you troubled because you do not get erections as easily as you used to?

YES → **Do you often fail to get an erection when you want to have sex or masturbate?**

YES → Most older men discover that they no longer get an erection as easily as they used to. You may find it easier at certain times than at others – in the afternoon, for example, rather than at night, when you are tired. But very frequent erection failure is not an inevitable consequence of old age. See the problem chart ERECTION PROBLEMS, p.36, for causes unrelated to aging.

NO ↓ (from "Do you often fail...")

A common symptom of aging is that you need more intense and prolonged stimulation of the penis in order to become fully aroused.

NO ↓ (from "Are you troubled...")

Do you worry because your erection is not as strong as it used to be?

YES → This is normal. You may find it easier to maintain a firm erection if your partner is on top or if she lies with a pillow beneath her buttocks. If you prefer a side-by-side position, she should move slightly lower down the bed once you are inside her, as your erection will be more easily maintained in this position.

NO ↓

Do you sometimes fail to ejaculate when you have intercourse?

YES → This is a natural consequence of aging. However, many men find that their ability to maintain an erection longer than when they were young is a considerable compensation for the occasional failure to reach a climax. Although you may not ejaculate every time, intercourse need be no less enjoyable than it was formerly.

NO ↓

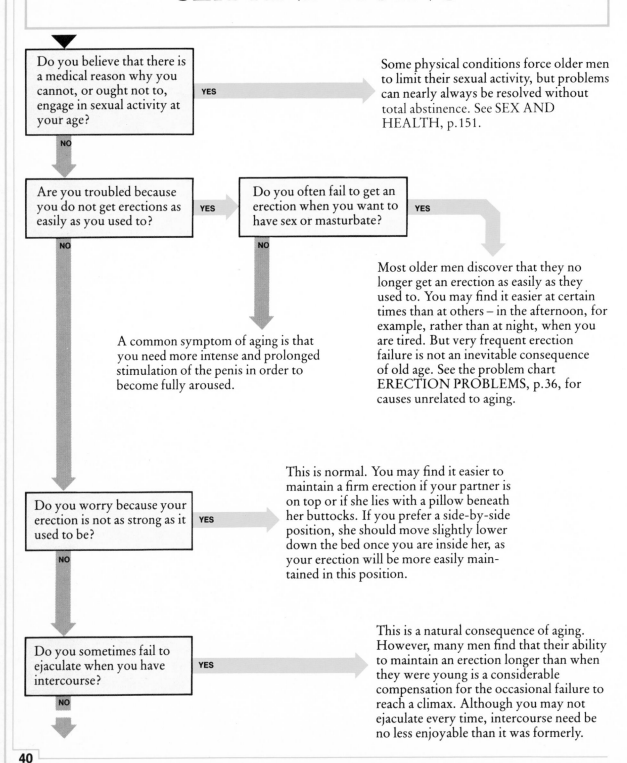

Is orgasm less intense than it used to be?

YES → Ejaculation generally becomes less powerful with age. Seminal fluid may seep out rather than spurt, and the feeling of inevitability that formerly preceded orgasm may diminish or disappear. These changes are no cause for concern.

NO ↓

Does it worry you that you have sex much less often than you used to?

YES → Masturbation is a short-term answer for the single man, whatever his age, but if you have a chance to establish a new partnership in later life, do not feel embarrassed about doing so. Old age does not necessarily signal the end of sexual desire, nor does it prevent the formation of emotional attachments involving sex.

NO ↓

Is this because you no longer have a full-time sexual partner?

YES →

NO ↓

Is it because you fear you are not fully satisfying your sexual partner?

YES → Age alone may not be the major cause of this problem, although it is often used as an honorable reason for failing to satisfy a partner in a relationship that has lost its edge. Both you and your partner will benefit from studying the fourth part of this book, THE MAN WITH A STEADY PARTNER.

NO ↓

Your sexual response may not be as intense in old age as in youth, but the capacity for enjoyment of sex can last into the seventies and even beyond. About one third of men in their late seventies are still sexually active and sexual decline is slower in those who have always had a full sex life.

SEX-HORMONE REPLACEMENT THERAPY

After the age of 60, production of the male sex hormone testosterone may fall to well below the 'normal' level. When this happens, there is a decline in sexual desire, with ejaculatory force being diminished. The ability to achieve erection is not affected, however. Some doctors have attempted to compensate with hormone replacement therapy, but the results have usually been disappointing.

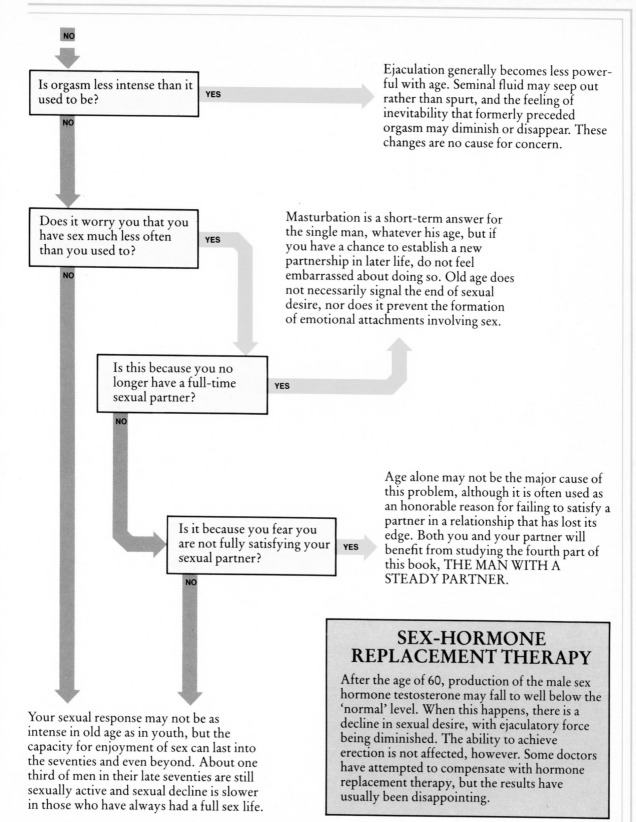

HETEROSEXUALITY/ HOMOSEXUALITY CONFLICTS

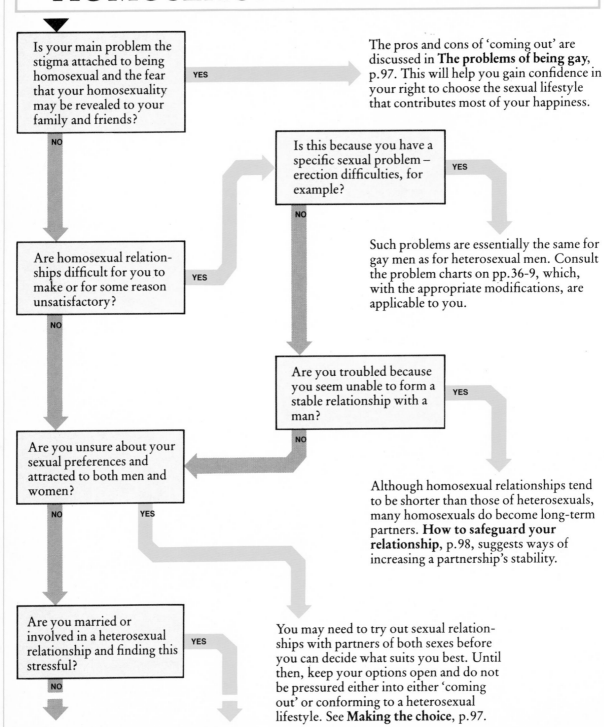

Is your main problem the stigma attached to being homosexual and the fear that your homosexuality may be revealed to your family and friends?

YES

The pros and cons of 'coming out' are discussed in **The problems of being gay**, p.97. This will help you gain confidence in your right to choose the sexual lifestyle that contributes most of your happiness.

NO

Are homosexual relationships difficult for you to make or for some reason unsatisfactory?

YES

Is this because you have a specific sexual problem – erection difficulties, for example?

YES

NO

Such problems are essentially the same for gay men as for heterosexual men. Consult the problem charts on pp.36-9, which, with the appropriate modifications, are applicable to you.

NO

Are you troubled because you seem unable to form a stable relationship with a man?

YES

Are you unsure about your sexual preferences and attracted to both men and women?

NO

Although homosexual relationships tend to be shorter than those of heterosexuals, many homosexuals do become long-term partners. **How to safeguard your relationship**, p.98, suggests ways of increasing a partnership's stability.

NO   **YES**

Are you married or involved in a heterosexual relationship and finding this stressful?

YES

You may need to try out sexual relationships with partners of both sexes before you can decide what suits you best. Until then, keep your options open and do not be pressured either into either 'coming out' or conforming to a heterosexual lifestyle. See **Making the choice**, p.97.

NO

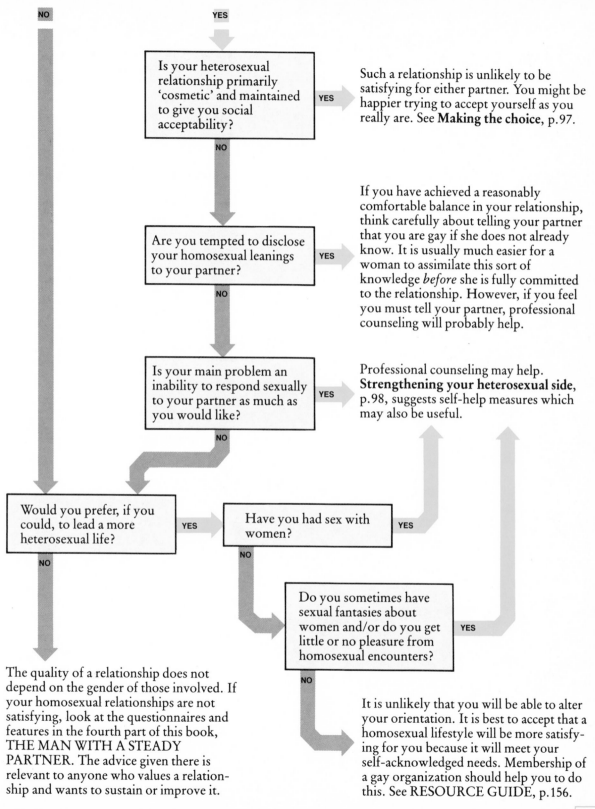

Is your heterosexual relationship primarily 'cosmetic' and maintained to give you social acceptability?

YES → Such a relationship is unlikely to be satisfying for either partner. You might be happier trying to accept yourself as you really are. See **Making the choice**, p.97.

Are you tempted to disclose your homosexual leanings to your partner?

YES → If you have achieved a reasonably comfortable balance in your relationship, think carefully about telling your partner that you are gay if she does not already know. It is usually much easier for a woman to assimilate this sort of knowledge *before* she is fully committed to the relationship. However, if you feel you must tell your partner, professional counseling will probably help.

Is your main problem an inability to respond sexually to your partner as much as you would like?

YES → Professional counseling may help. **Strengthening your heterosexual side**, p.98, suggests self-help measures which may also be useful.

Would you prefer, if you could, to lead a more heterosexual life?

YES → **Have you had sex with women?**

YES →

NO →

Do you sometimes have sexual fantasies about women and/or do you get little or no pleasure from homosexual encounters?

YES →

NO →

The quality of a relationship does not depend on the gender of those involved. If your homosexual relationships are not satisfying, look at the questionnaires and features in the fourth part of this book, THE MAN WITH A STEADY PARTNER. The advice given there is relevant to anyone who values a relationship and wants to sustain or improve it.

It is unlikely that you will be able to alter your orientation. It is best to accept that a homosexual lifestyle will be more satisfying for you because it will meet your self-acknowledged needs. Membership of a gay organization should help you to do this. See RESOURCE GUIDE, p.156.

GENDER PROBLEMS

Is your only problem that you sometimes find it difficult to live up to the traditional male role, or feel you would like to develop your feminine side a little?

YES → The 'macho' image is not one that many women find particularly attractive. In fact they often value the traditionally feminine qualities – tenderness, warmth, the ability to show feelings – much more. See **What makes a good lover?**, p.48.

NO

Do you occasionally enjoy dressing as a woman?

YES → At such times do you wear make-up and behave as much like a woman as possible?

YES → Is this because you find it sexually arousing to wear women's clothes?

NO

Do you sometimes have homosexual relationships simply because they seem easier and less threatening than heterosexual ones?

NO

Is it because you feel more relaxed and comfortable dressed as a woman?

YES

YES

These are indications of transvestism, which is discussed on p.100.

This does not mean that you are homosexual, but that you do not yet have the confidence in your own masculinity to make relationships with women. See **Dispelling sexual anxiety**, p.69.

NO

Is it because you feel you really *are* a woman, despite a male body and genitals?

YES

NO

You probably just enjoy cross-dressing for fun or as a defiant gesture because it is taboo. It does not necessarily follow that you have a gender problem.

Do men attract you sexually more than women?

NO   **YES**

This tendency, transsexualism, is discussed on p.101.

Your ability to feel masculine depends in part on your sexual self-esteem. If this is low, you are sure to have doubts about yourself. IMPROVING YOUR SELF-ESTEEM, p.71, should help you feel more confident of your masculinity.

If you have recently 'come out' as a homosexual you may enjoy being exaggeratedly effeminate for a while. Once you feel at home in your new role, however, this tendency and the urge to cross-dress will probably disappear.

UNUSUAL SEXUAL PRACTICES

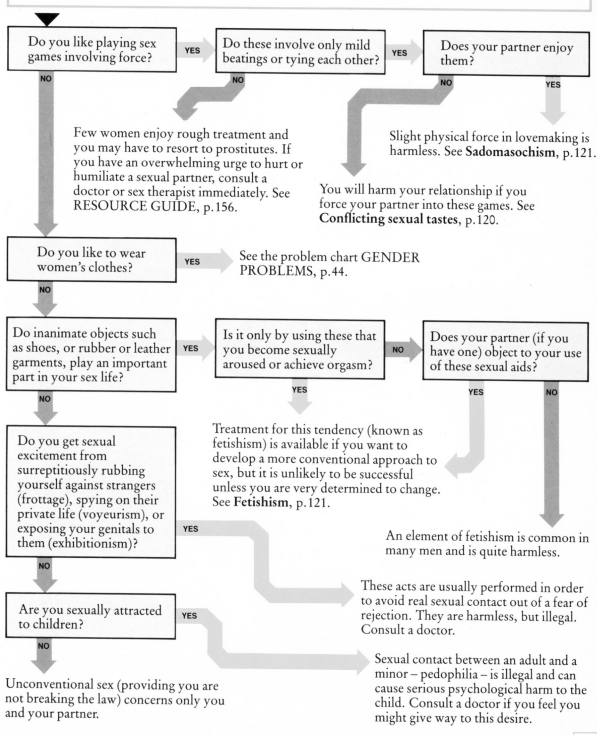

Do you like playing sex games involving force? **YES**

Do these involve only mild beatings or tying each other? **YES**

Does your partner enjoy them? **NO** **YES**

NO

Few women enjoy rough treatment and you may have to resort to prostitutes. If you have an overwhelming urge to hurt or humiliate a sexual partner, consult a doctor or sex therapist immediately. See RESOURCE GUIDE, p.156.

Slight physical force in lovemaking is harmless. See **Sadomasochism**, p.121.

You will harm your relationship if you force your partner into these games. See **Conflicting sexual tastes**, p.120.

Do you like to wear women's clothes? **YES**

See the problem chart GENDER PROBLEMS, p.44.

NO

Do inanimate objects such as shoes, or rubber or leather garments, play an important part in your sex life? **YES**

Is it only by using these that you become sexually aroused or achieve orgasm? **NO**

Does your partner (if you have one) object to your use of these sexual aids? **YES** **NO**

NO **YES**

Do you get sexual excitement from surreptitiously rubbing yourself against strangers (frottage), spying on their private life (voyeurism), or exposing your genitals to them (exhibitionism)? **YES**

Treatment for this tendency (known as fetishism) is available if you want to develop a more conventional approach to sex, but it is unlikely to be successful unless you are very determined to change. See **Fetishism**, p.121.

An element of fetishism is common in many men and is quite harmless.

NO

Are you sexually attracted to children? **YES**

These acts are usually performed in order to avoid real sexual contact out of a fear of rejection. They are harmless, but illegal. Consult a doctor.

NO

Sexual contact between an adult and a minor – pedophilia – is illegal and can cause serious psychological harm to the child. Consult a doctor if you feel you might give way to this desire.

Unconventional sex (providing you are not breaking the law) concerns only you and your partner.

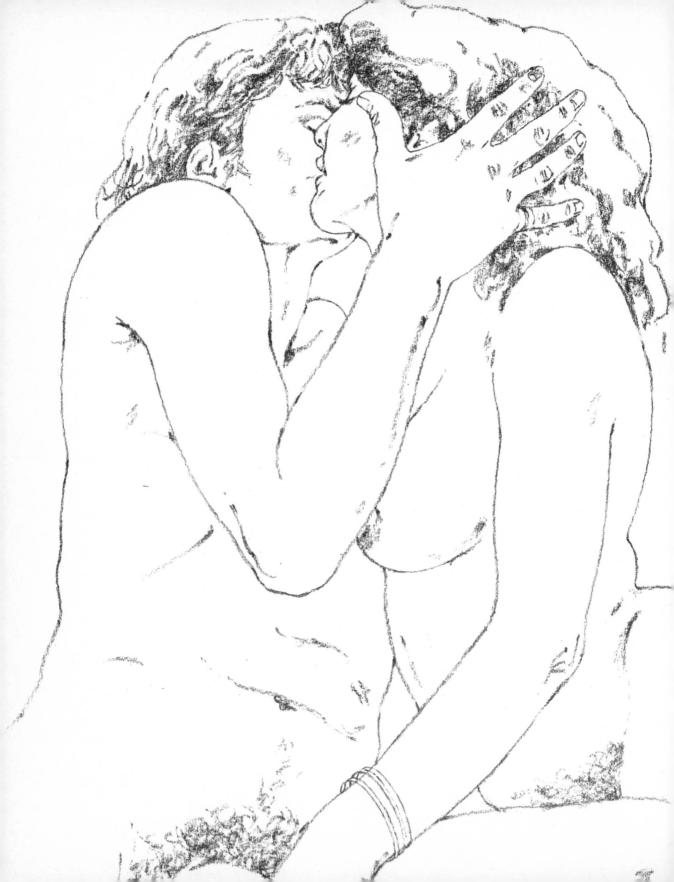

3

IMPROVING YOUR SEX LIFE

The aim of this part of the book is to help you develop
your full sexual potential, discover ways of enhancing and
sustaining a good sex life, and derive more enjoyment if it
is currently unsatisfying. The advice given is relevant to
any man, married or single, regardless of age or experience.
However good your sex life, it can be fun to try something
new, to experiment a little. This helps to keep your interest
in each other alive, and ensures that your relationship will
continue to be as sensual as it ever was. There is never a
need to feel too old, or that you have been together too
long, to make any changes. It is even possible that you may
get more pleasure from the activities suggested than you
would have done when you were younger and less sure of
yourself and your partner.
This section also deals with some of the difficulties that
take the edge off sexual enjoyment. However longstanding
a sexual problem is, do not feel that it is too late to try to
resolve it. You will experience a marked improvement in
your sex life, or overcome your problems altogether, if you
follow the self-help programs.

EXPANDING YOUR SEXUAL REPERTOIRE

In recent years, many surveys have revealed that women are largely in accord as to their sexual likes and dislikes. What has emerged most clearly is that many no longer want the strong, silent, 'macho' male. Instead, they value the man who can make them feel good emotionally as well as physically.

What makes a good lover?

While a large part of being a good lover lies in the ability to satisfy your partner's emotional needs, you also need to keep the relationship exciting by exploring a range of sexual activities. Below you will discover techniques to make your sex life less routine. But first, some pointers to becoming a more sensitive lover.

☐ Be sensual as well as sexual. For most women, the caresses of foreplay, which you may see simply as a way of 'priming' your partner for sex, can be as enjoyable as intercourse itself.

☐ Use touch to show affection, as well as to ask for sex. A hug or a kiss need not just be a prelude to bed but can show simply that you care for her.

☐ Do not be afraid to let your arousal wane during sex and to relax and talk a while.

☐ Remember that afterplay matters as much as foreplay. You need not do much, but a cuddle and a few loving words are essential. Never roll over and go straight to sleep, or leap out of bed and get dressed.

☐ Do not approach a new sexual activity as a challenge – something designed to test you – but as a possible source of pleasure. The only real failure is not enjoying what you are doing. But be guided by instinct. An experience is not necessarily good because it is new. If you are not drawn to something, do not try it. If you do it and dislike it, do not repeat it.

☐ If sex has always seemed something of a disappointment, it probably will not help much just to widen your repertoire. Sex can provide only a limited range of sensations, and what takes it beyond the predictable for most people is the quality of the relationship involved.

☐ Women can accept an occasional failure, and it may even make you more human, vulnerable, and easy to love. If you feel obliged to be constantly ready for sex, you will take the inevitable occasional failure too hard.

ASSESSING YOUR SEXUAL REPERTOIRE

The checklist on the right will help you determine the scope of your sexual experience and, because it may include possibilities that you think would be fun but have never tried, will widen your horizons. It also gives you a chance to judge the degree of pleasure you are currently getting from sex and to test the balance of giving and receiving between you and your steady partner (if you have one). If your preferences include things you enjoy doing for a partner as well as things you like to have done for you, you are more likely than not to be able to maintain a satisfactory relationship.

On a 0–4 scale, indicate in the columns provided: first, how much you enjoy the activity, and, secondly, how often you do it. The list is highly selective, so feel free to add other activities you perform that are not included.

Checking your ratings

Ideally you should find that activities to which you have assigned a high enjoyment rating also have a high frequency rating. If not, ask yourself why not. On the other hand, if there are any activities to which you have assigned a higher rating for frequency for than for enjoyment, give some serious thought to the question of why this is so. Are you doing something you do not particularly like chiefly to please your partner? If so, this is a healthy attitude – but only up to a point. The frequent practice of any activity that you dislike may not only cause resentment but could lead to erection difficulties.

A balanced relationship

Why not study the above list together so as to consider how well your responses match each other?

Items 2, 6, 8, 10, 12, 14, 22, and 24 are things you can do to arouse and please your partner. Items 3, 7, 9, 11, 13, 15, 23, and 25 are things your partner can do to you. Your frequency ratings and levels of enjoyment for each of these two sets of activities should be similar, if not exactly the same.

If they are not, what is the reason? Does one of you tend to be the giver, the other the recipient of pleasure? If this is the case, you will probably both find a better balance between your roles more fulfilling. You might also consider activities which you feel you would enjoy very much, but which, for some reason, you have never tried. These, of course, would attract a high enjoyment rating but nil for frequency. Having acknowledged your lack of fulfilment in these areas, you need to share your problems with your partner, particularly if it is her reluctance that has prevented experimentation.

ENJOYMENT RATING					FREQUENCY RATING				
Very high 4		Low 1			Regularly 4		Seldom 1		
High 3		Nil 0			Often 3		Never 0		
Medium 2					Sometimes 2				
		ENJOY-MENT	FRE-QUENCY				ENJOY-MENT	FRE-QUENCY	
1 'French kissing' (tongues in each other's mouths).					**14** Giving your partner an orgasm by manual stimulation.				
2 'Petting' (fondling your partner's clothed body).					**15** Being manually stimulated to orgasm by your partner.				
3 Having your partner fondle your clothed body.					**16** Having intercourse in a man-on-top position.				
4 Seeing your partner naked.					**17** Or with your partner on top.				
5 Being seen naked.					**18** Or in a side-by-side position.				
6 Caressing your partner's naked body.					**19** Having intercourse in a rear-entry position.				
7 Having yours caressed.					**20** Or in a sitting position.				
8 Kissing your partner's breasts and sucking the nipples.					**21** Having intercourse in a standing position.				
9 Having your partner kiss and suck your nipples.					**22** Fondling or kissing your partner's buttocks and anus.				
10 Exploring and stroking your partner's genitals.					**23** Having your buttocks and anus fondled or kissed.				
11 Having your partner explore and stroke your genitals.					**24** Using oral stimulation to bring your partner to orgasm.				
12 Licking and kissing your partner's genitals.					**25** Being brought to orgasm by oral stimulation.				
13 Having yours kissed.									

STIMULATION TECHNIQUES

The stimulation techniques or foreplay described here are used by most couples to arouse each other, but they need not always lead to intercourse. They are in themselves valuable as a source of pleasure.

Clitoral stimulation

Stimulation of the clitoris, the method most women use for masturbation, is probably the most effective way of arousing a woman and the easiest way for many women to reach orgasm. It is, however, a technique at which, according to surveys of American women, most men are not very skilful.

Your partner, knowing her own body and its reactions, can show you the precise spot, the pressure, and the rhythm that excite her most. So ask her to guide your hand at first if you have not tried clitoral stimulation before. If she is too inexperienced or inhibited to help you in this way, you will have to experiment. The following guidelines should help

you, but you will certainly get further more quickly if you can talk freely to each other.

___

☐ Be gentle when you touch the clitoris as it is a delicate and sensitive organ. A lubricant – for example, your partner's vaginal fluid, your own saliva, or a commercial preparation – will minimize irritation.

___

☐ Do not use direct or sustained pressure on the clitoris unless you are sure your partner likes it; many women find it irritating or even painful. Indirect pressure through the folds of flesh around the clitoris is generally both more comfortable and more stimulating. Use your whole hand, all the fingers, the palm, or the heel of the hand, rather than just one or two fingers. This spreads a subtle but highly satisfying pressure over the entire highly responsive clitoral area.

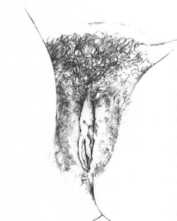

◁ **The female genitals**
The external female genitals are known as the vulva. On arousal the vaginal lips fill with blood and cushion the orifice. The outer lips, the labia majora, vary in shape and color, while the inner pair, the labia minora, are generally pinker and moister.

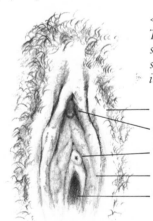

◁ **The clitoris**
This small, highly sensitive organ is situated within the inner vaginal lips.

— LABIA MAJORA

— CLITORIS

— URETHRAL ORIFICE

— LABIA MINORA

— VAGINAL ORIFICE

CLITORAL STIMULATION TECHNIQUES

Individual preferences vary enormously, but at least one of the methods described below should work for your partner.

1 CIRCULAR MOVEMENTS

1 Place your hand over the clitoral area, applying light pressure with your fingers or palm, and move it gently round and round.

2 Move it up so that the heel is at the top of the vulva, right over the clitoris. Your hand should be resting partly on the pubic bone on either side. In this position you can press quite firmly as you rub.

3 Alternatively, you can put your hand, palm downward, over the pubic mound so that your fingers overhang the clitoral area. Pressing gently, make firm, circular movements.

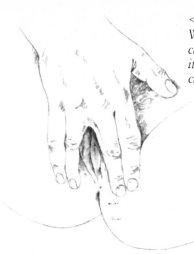

◁ **Using the heel of the hand**
With the heel of your hand on the clitoris and the pubic bone either side of it, apply firm pressure while making a circular rubbing movement.

Rotating the palm ▷
You can give firm but gentle circular stimulation to the whole clitoral area when the palm of your hand covers the pubic mound and the fingers hang down.

2 VIBRATORY MOVEMENTS

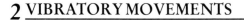

1 Cup your hand over the whole area and vibrate it rapidly.

2 Brush your fingers rapidly to and fro across the clitoris.

3 With your hand resting on the pubic mound, put a finger each side of the vaginal lips and vibrate them from side to side.

4 Rub on each side of the inner vaginal lips at the base of the clitoris. Because you are applying pressure through the fleshy folds rather than directly to the clitoris, you can press quite firmly.

5 An effective alternative is a combination of clitoral stimulation with digital penetration of the vagina (make sure that your fingernail has no jagged edges). Using your right hand, palm upward, slip your middle finger into the vagina. Your other fingers should be bent forward so that the knuckles press against the clitoral area.

6 Move the finger gently in and out, pressing on the front wall of the vagina, so stimulating an especially sensitive area (known as the G spot). This internal vaginal pressure, combined with friction on the clitoris, is intensely pleasurable.

7 Rubbing the tip of the penis against the clitoris is perhaps the best means of arousal.

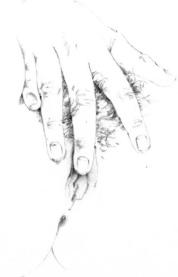

◁ **Brushing with the fingers**
The simplest method of stimulating the clitoris with a vibratory action is to brush your fingers rapidly back and forth against it.

Stimulating the G spot ▷
While you use your middle finger to explore the front wall of the vagina, with its highly sensitive G spot, your knuckles can stimulate the clitoris indirectly by pressing on the surrounding area.

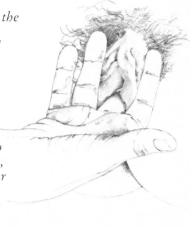

ORAL SEX

Stimulation of the male genitals with the mouth is known as fellatio, corresponding stimulation of the female genitals as cunnilingus. Both are fairly safe activities as far as the transmission of AIDS is concerned (see **Guidelines for safer sex**, p.154).

Most men enjoy both giving and receiving oral sex. Some, however, would like to try it but hesitate to mention it to their partner, feeling that it is abnormal or something to be ashamed of. Others avoid it because they dislike genital odors and secretions (see **Anxiety about sexual odors and secretions,** p. 70).

Oral stimulation ▷
The '69' position allows mutual oral-genital contact and can be intensely exciting. Many couples, however, prefer to take turns in giving each other oral stimulation, as it is easier to concentrate on either giving or receiving pleasure than to do both simultaneously.

Fellatio

Many women, even if they are happy to try oral sex, are unsure of exactly what to do. Try to be as explicit as you can when you tell your partner what you would like. At first it is probably best just to suggest that she kisses your penis until she feels more comfortable with the idea of taking it into her mouth.

She will probably soon want to take the whole head inside her mouth and suck it, using her tongue to play on the sensitive underside ridge, or frenulum. She will need to open her mouth wide and close her lips (but not her teeth) firmly around the head.

Then she can move her mouth up and down on your penis, just as you would move it in her vagina. She can make an extension of her mouth by encircling your penis with her thumb and forefinger, moving mouth and hand up and down on it in the same rhythm. You can guide her head with your hands to indicate the pace you prefer but be careful not to force her movements.

As she becomes more confident she will probably take more of the shaft into her mouth, and you will want to thrust lightly. Remember, though, that she may not be able to let your penis touch the back of her throat without gagging, and so you should allow her to control the depth of your thrusts.

When such inhibitions are overcome, oral sex is usually highly enjoyable for both partners.

You can use oral stimulation to arouse each other before intercourse, or as an alternative means of reaching orgasm. But you should avoid it if either of you has an infection of the mouth or the genitals.

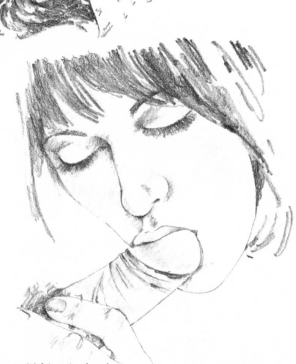

△ **Taking it slowly**
If your partner has never sucked your penis before, she will probably prefer just to kiss or lick it at first.

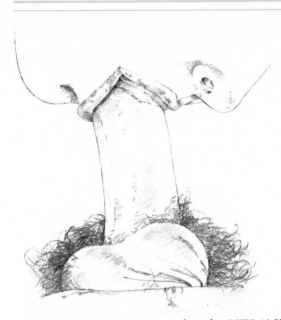

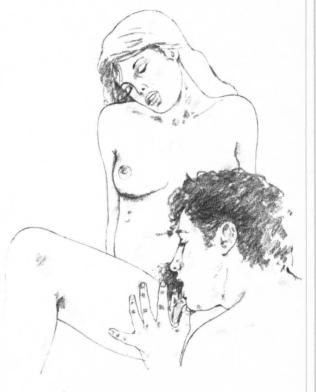

Current evidence suggests that the HIV (AIDS) virus is probably not transmitted during oral sex, possibly because saliva contains a substance which inactivates the virus. However, someone who has mouth sores, a mouth infection or bleeding gums (which are all quite common) may be at risk if an infected partner ejaculates in their mouth. Use of a condom during oral sex will prevent infection (see **Guidelines for safer sex**, p.154).

Cunnilingus

Since the tongue is softer than the fingers, it can be used to provide gentler stimulation of the clitoris. Your partner will probably find cunnilingus extremely satisfying, as long as she feels you too are enjoying it. Nothing detracts from a woman's pleasure in oral sex as much as a suspicion that it is being done dutifully, out of consideration for her. The following advice should help you give your partner maximum pleasure.

Begin by kissing and licking the pubic mound, the inner side of the thighs, and the lower belly. Now move your tongue over the genital area, flicking it along the fleshy folds up to the clitoris. Note your partner's responses, and act accordingly.

Gently probe the clitoris with your tongue. Again, discover from her reactions the kind of stimulation that your partner most enjoys. Begin by simply nuzzling and sucking. You may also find it exciting to vibrate your tongue rapidly against the clitoris.

Use your hands, too – to caress her breasts, stroke her thighs, or hold her buttocks firmly. Such gestures bring an additional closeness that is easily overlooked during cunnilingus.

△ **Fear of choking**
Your partner can allay any anxiety she might have about choking by encircling the penis with one or more fingers to limit penetration. Remind her to keep her teeth clear of the particularly sensitive head of your penis (left).

△ **Arousing your partner**
Kissing the area around your partner's vaginal entrance will sharpen her anticipation as well as providing indirect but intense stimulation of the clitoris.

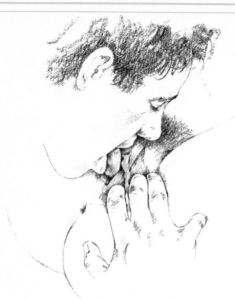

△ **Penetration with the tongue**
Thrusting your tongue in and out of the entrance to the vagina may prove highly arousing for your partner. But some women prefer attention to the clitoris.

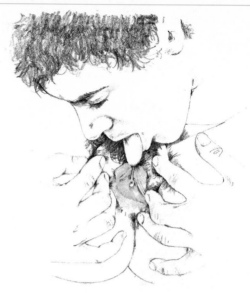

△ **Using the tip of the tongue**
By separating the vaginal lips and holding them open gently with both hands, you can flick the tip of your tongue over the exposed clitoris.

ANAL SEX

The most basic form of anal stimulation is known as postillionage, which means touching the partner's anus during intercourse or oral sex. The anal area is very sensitive, and postillionage can intensify erotic sensations greatly.

Penetration of the rectum by a section or all of the finger is a more advanced version of the technique. If you and your partner want to do this, use some lubrication on the finger, and make sure there are no jagged fingernails. If she slips her finger a couple of inches inside your rectum and exerts pressure forward on your prostate gland, you will experience intense excitement.

Anal intercourse – penis in rectum – is primarily a homosexual activity, but a substantial minority of heterosexual couples occasionally practice it. However, because the lining of the rectum is thin, delicate and easily damaged, the HIV (AIDS) virus is more easily transmitted during anal intercourse than during any other form of sexual activity. The inserter should always wear a strong condom and use plenty of a spermicide or lubricant containing nonoxynol-9, which has been shown to kill the HIV virus. Penetration can be painful, so make it slow and gentle. Stop immediately if your partner asks you to. If your partner is on top, she can control entry and depth of penetration.

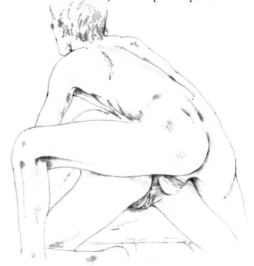

△ **Hygienic precautions**
Never have vaginal intercourse after anal without washing your penis well, or you both risk genital infection.

SEXUAL POSITIONS

There are six basic groups of positions for intercourse, within which there are innumerable variations that differ only in minor details such as the relative position of your limbs or the angle of your bodies to one another. Many of the examples selected for the following pages combine a high degree of stimulation with comfort.

Some of the positions are especially appropriate for particular situations – during pregnancy, for example. Others are strictly for fun, with no special value except that of novelty, but you may find them worth trying on occasion.

The value of experimentation
Do not feel you have to go entirely by the book when you try a new position. If it feels awkward, make small adjustments until it is right for both of you. You will probably find that, no matter how many of them you try, you will keep coming back to the few that give you and your partner the most mutual pleasure.

If you prefer this approach, it does not mean that you are unadventurous, but that you have experimented enough to know what you like. (The obvious time for experimentation is at the beginning of a new relationship when you want to explore each other's bodies and search out each other's preferences. It is also useful after you have been together a long time and want to enliven your lovemaking by trying something new.)

Remember that:

- ☐ Penetration is easiest if your partner's thighs are widely spread.

- ☐ Positions in which your partner's knees are bent up to her chest allow for deepest penetration.

- ☐ A position in which your partner's legs are held together provides maximum stimulation for the penis.

MAN-ON-TOP POSITIONS

The man-on-top positions, and in particular the 'missionary', in which the man lies between the woman's slightly parted legs, are probably the most widely used group of positions. They give you almost total control over intercourse, but allow your partner very little freedom of movement. These positions are, for most men, the easiest in which to reach orgasm.

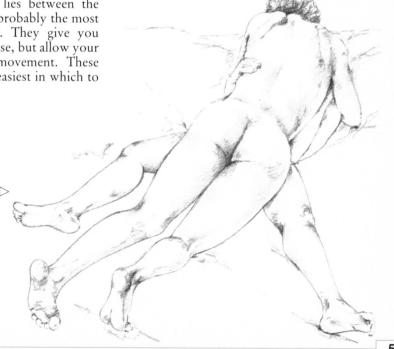

Deep penetration with intense stimulation of clitoris and penis ▷
In this position, the vulva faces downward to a greater degree than in the more common knees-flexed postures, providing extra stimulation for the clitoris. Penetration is deep and the entrance to the vagina is narrowed, so that the penis also receives considerable stimulation.

Compensating for a short penis ▷
This deep-penetration position is useful if the penis is short. The vaginal opening is slack, but the clitoris receives good stimulation and the woman is able to move in rhythm with her partner.

▽ **'Split-level' position**
In this 'split-level' position the woman lies on the bed and the man stands or kneels beside it. By lifting her, he can alter the angle of penetration.

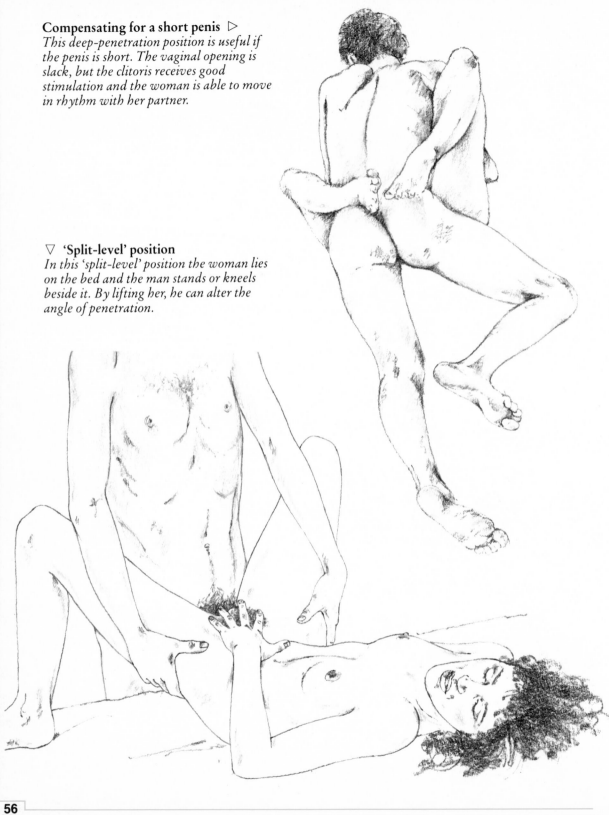

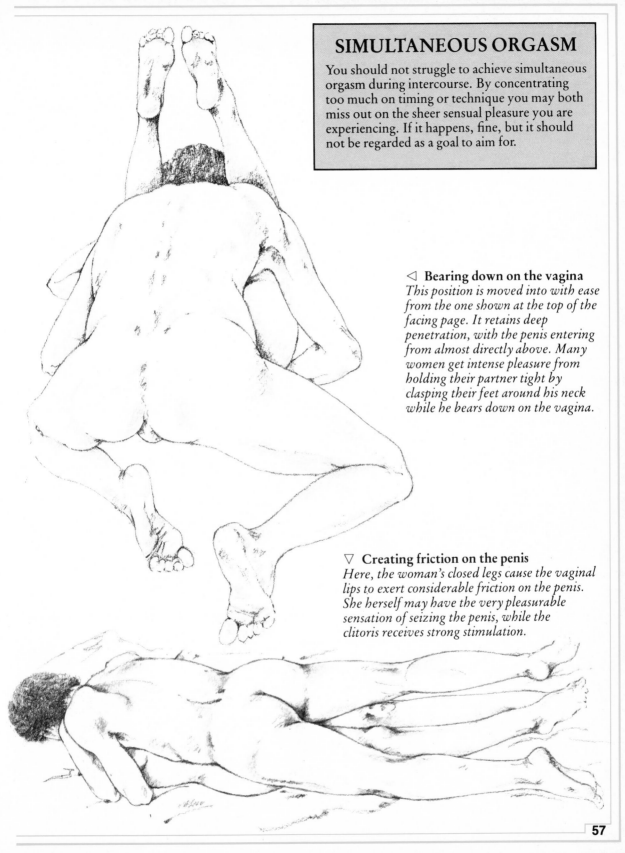

SIMULTANEOUS ORGASM

You should not struggle to achieve simultaneous orgasm during intercourse. By concentrating too much on timing or technique you may both miss out on the sheer sensual pleasure you are experiencing. If it happens, fine, but it should not be regarded as a goal to aim for.

◁ **Bearing down on the vagina**
This position is moved into with ease from the one shown at the top of the facing page. It retains deep penetration, with the penis entering from almost directly above. Many women get intense pleasure from holding their partner tight by clasping their feet around his neck while he bears down on the vagina.

▽ **Creating friction on the penis**
Here, the woman's closed legs cause the vaginal lips to exert considerable friction on the penis. She herself may have the very pleasurable sensation of seizing the penis, while the clitoris receives strong stimulation.

WOMAN-ON-TOP POSITIONS

Many couples find the woman-on-top positions particularly satisfying. They give your partner a chance to make love to you, allowing her to control both depth of penetration, which can be helpful if she is apprehensive through lack of experience, and the tempo of lovemaking. These positions are good if you are much heavier or if she is pregnant.

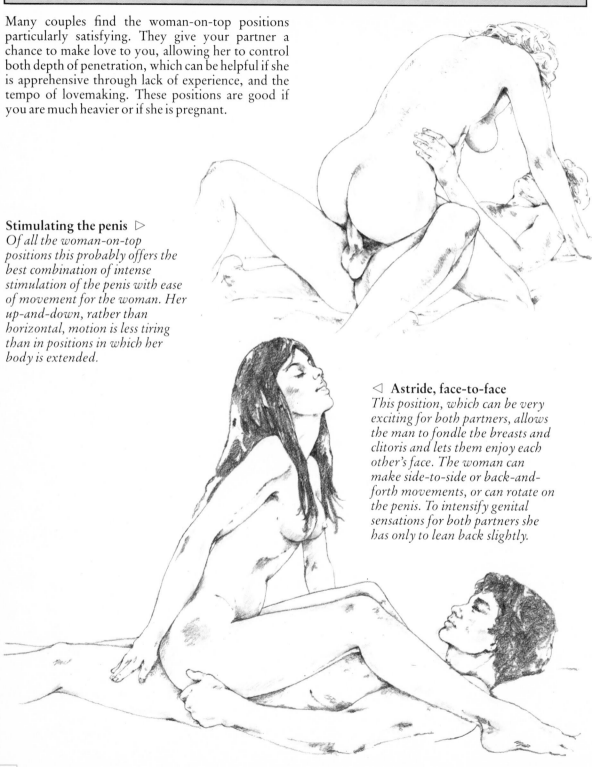

Stimulating the penis ▷
Of all the woman-on-top positions this probably offers the best combination of intense stimulation of the penis with ease of movement for the woman. Her up-and-down, rather than horizontal, motion is less tiring than in positions in which her body is extended.

◁ **Astride, face-to-face**
This position, which can be very exciting for both partners, allows the man to fondle the breasts and clitoris and lets them enjoy each other's face. The woman can make side-to-side or back-and-forth movements, or can rotate on the penis. To intensify genital sensations for both partners she has only to lean back slightly.

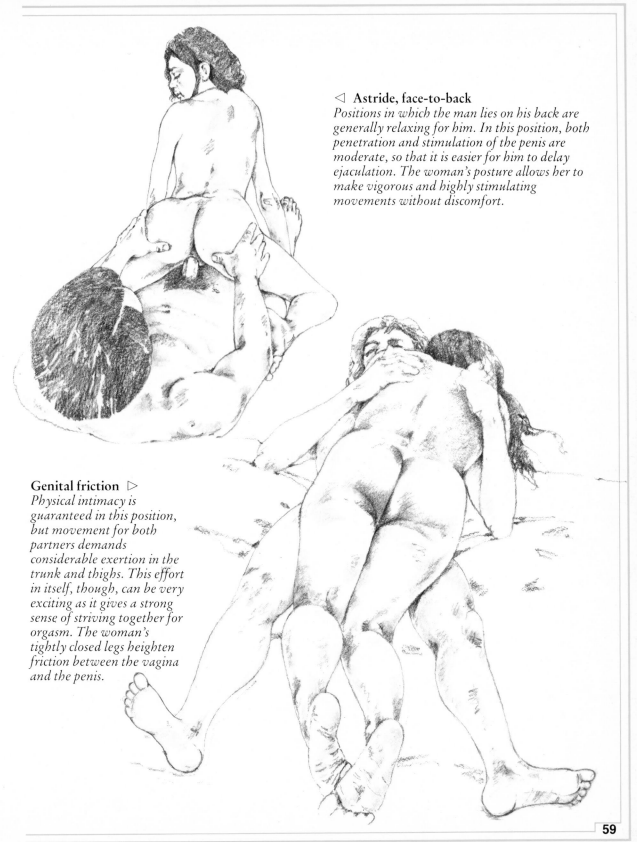

◁ **Astride, face-to-back**
Positions in which the man lies on his back are generally relaxing for him. In this position, both penetration and stimulation of the penis are moderate, so that it is easier for him to delay ejaculation. The woman's posture allows her to make vigorous and highly stimulating movements without discomfort.

Genital friction ▷
Physical intimacy is guaranteed in this position, but movement for both partners demands considerable exertion in the trunk and thighs. This effort in itself, though, can be very exciting as it gives a strong sense of striving together for orgasm. The woman's tightly closed legs heighten friction between the vagina and the penis.

REAR-ENTRY POSITIONS

This group of positions allows penetration while lying, standing, sitting, kneeling, or with the woman on top. In most of these positions the woman does not bear the man's weight and so has considerable freedom to move during intercourse. Most offer the advantage that you can fondle your partner's breasts and clitoris at the same time and nearly all are comfortable when she is in late pregnancy.

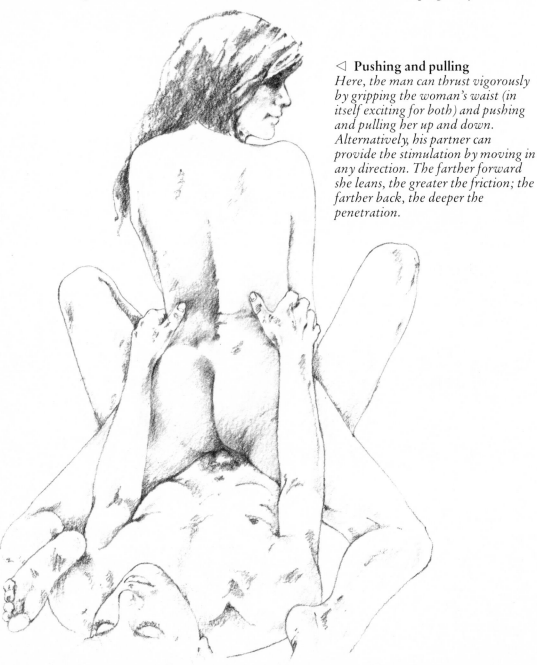

◁ **Pushing and pulling**
Here, the man can thrust vigorously by gripping the woman's waist (in itself exciting for both) and pushing and pulling her up and down. Alternatively, his partner can provide the stimulation by moving in any direction. The farther forward she leans, the greater the friction; the farther back, the deeper the penetration.

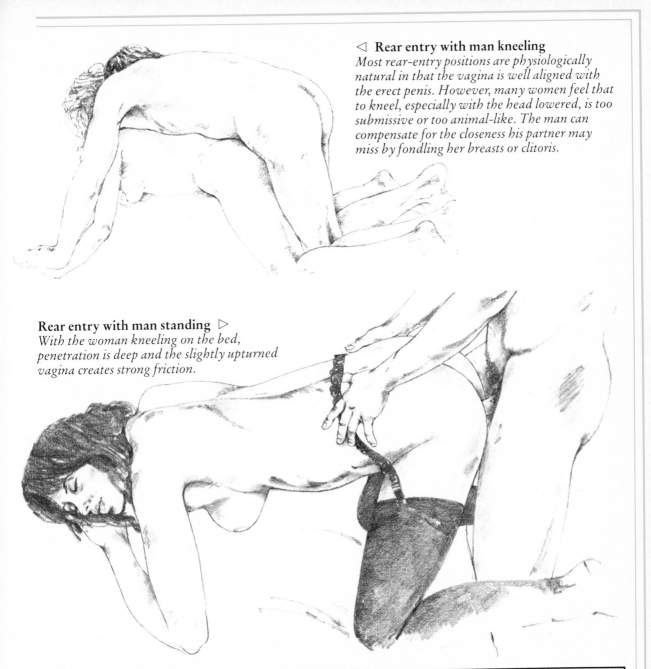

◁ **Rear entry with man kneeling**
Most rear-entry positions are physiologically natural in that the vagina is well aligned with the erect penis. However, many women feel that to kneel, especially with the head lowered, is too submissive or too animal-like. The man can compensate for the closeness his partner may miss by fondling her breasts or clitoris.

Rear entry with man standing ▷
With the woman kneeling on the bed, penetration is deep and the slightly upturned vagina creates strong friction.

G-SPOT STIMULATION

The vagina is not overall a very sensitive organ, but it does have two particularly sensitive spots: the entrance, and a small area, known as the Graffenburg or G spot, about halfway up the front wall. Many women find that pressure on this area produces orgasm.

The G spot is stimulated in any position in which the penis presses against the front vaginal wall. The ones that are best will depend on the particular 'fit' of you and your partner(see SEXUAL POSITIONS, p.55). G-spot stimulation in man-on-top positions is increased by putting a pillow under your partner's hips.

SIDE-BY-SIDE POSITIONS

For relaxed, unhurried lovemaking, side-by-side positions are ideal, and couples often fall comfortably asleep locked together after making love this way. Side-by-side intercourse works well in pregnancy too, or if either of you is very heavy. A drawback for the woman is that her clitoris gets little stimulation from the pressure of your body, but in some variants it can be stimulated manually.

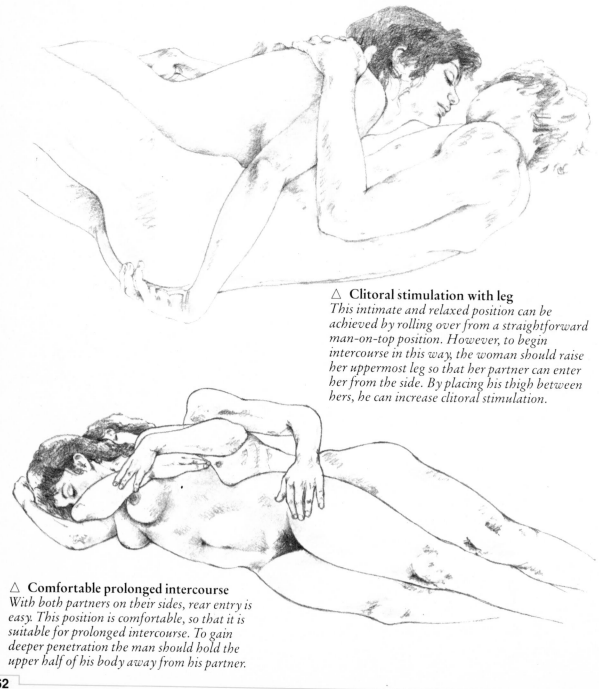

△ **Clitoral stimulation with leg**
This intimate and relaxed position can be achieved by rolling over from a straightforward man-on-top position. However, to begin intercourse in this way, the woman should raise her uppermost leg so that her partner can enter her from the side. By placing his thigh between hers, he can increase clitoral stimulation.

△ **Comfortable prolonged intercourse**
With both partners on their sides, rear entry is easy. This position is comfortable, so that it is suitable for prolonged intercourse. To gain deeper penetration the man should hold the upper half of his body away from his partner.

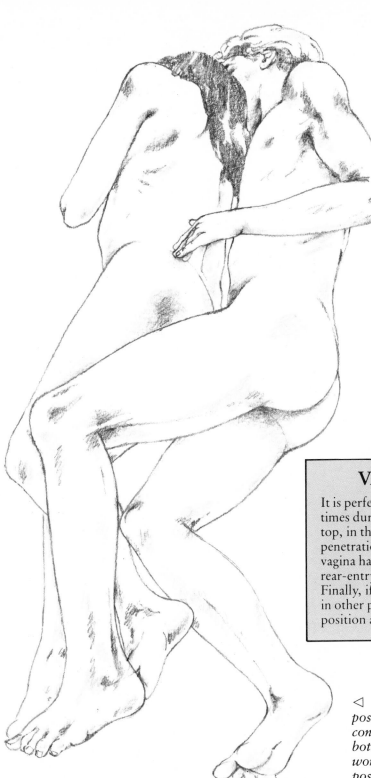

MULTIPLE ORGASMS

A few men say that they are capable of having multiple orgasms during intercourse, with all the normal intense and pleasurable sensations, but without ejaculation, and without losing their erection. Intercourse culminates in one final, very intense, orgasm which is simultaneous with ejaculation.

VARYING POSITION

It is perfectly natural to change positions several times during intercourse. You might start on top, in the most convenient position for easy penetration, and then, after your partner's vagina has had a while to relax, move into a rear-entry or deep-penetration position. Finally, if you find it difficult to have an orgasm in other positions, return to a man-on-top position as your climax approaches.

◁ **Relaxed intimacy** *The 'spoons' position gives a relaxed closeness and considerable freedom of movement for both partners. Absence of pressure on the woman from the man's weight makes this position particularly suitable when she is in late pregnancy.*

SITTING POSITIONS

Although few of the sitting positions allow you much movement or direct genital stimulation, many couples find them erotic, partly because of their novelty and partly because they provide a strong sense of intimacy. They are also restful positions that can be used when you want intercourse again after a tiring first bout.

Sitting, woman astride ▷
Sitting positions in which the couple face each other are psychologically stimulating and strong on novelty, if somewhat restrictive of movement. But, by stretching his arms out behind him to support himself, the man can thrust or at least make it easier for the woman to move on his penis.

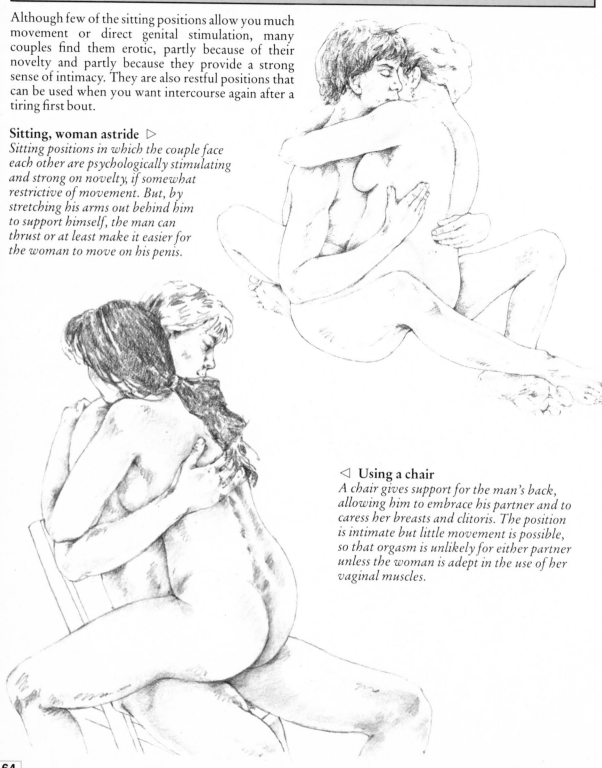

◁ **Using a chair**
A chair gives support for the man's back, allowing him to embrace his partner and to caress her breasts and clitoris. The position is intimate but little movement is possible, so that orgasm is unlikely for either partner unless the woman is adept in the use of her vaginal muscles.

STANDING POSITIONS

As with the sitting positions, the main benefit here is novelty. However, penetration is often difficult, especially if you are much taller than your partner, and she may need to stand on something in order to effect it.

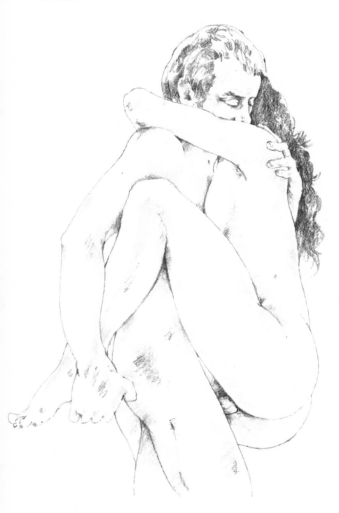

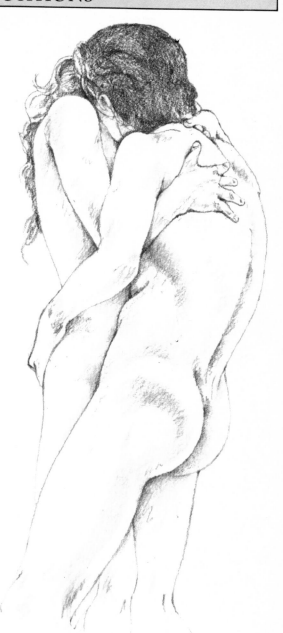

△ **Supporting the woman**
Considerable agility and strength are required in this position and it is likely to be no more than a brief variant of the position shown on the right. The man can support his partner as shown here, if she is light, or by placing one or both hands under her buttocks.

△ **Basic standing position**
This is the simplest standing position, often used when a couple want to dispense with the preliminaries. In order to keep the penis from slipping out, the woman usually needs to close her legs. If the man wants to thrust vigorously his partner can use a wall for support.

INCREASING YOUR PLEASURE

The following checklist suggests activities you and your partner might try if you want to introduce some novelty into a relationship which has become slightly stale. These are not necessarily things you will want to do often, however much you enjoy them. They are meant to introduce variety into a sexual routine, not simply to become part of that routine, for used too often they easily lose their stimulus.

You may not like all the ideas suggested. For example, although some men find it very exciting to share their sexual fantasies with their partner, others would consider this an intolerable invasion of privacy. Use your own judgement, and regard this list as merely a starting point to stimulate your imagination. As with any form of sexual activity, all that really matters is that you should both enjoy what you do.

☐ Take a bath or shower together.

☐ Make love in the dark (if you usually prefer some light) and vice versa.

☐ Make love somewhere other than the bed – on a chair, sofa, or rug, perhaps.

☐ Make love at an unusual time. Come home from work at lunchtime, for example.

☐ Use a mirror to watch yourselves making love.

☐ Make love outdoors, but be careful to choose a place where you will not be interrupted.

☐ Create a sensual atmosphere with music and candlelight.

☐ Combine lovemaking with a snack and a bottle of wine in bed.

☐ Read an erotic novel or poetry to each other in bed, or watch a sexy video together.

☐ Give each other a sensual and relaxing overall massage with scented body oils. Also, use feathers, velvet, fur, and other textures to give a variety of sensations to the skin.

☐ Tell your partner your favorite fantasy. If your own fantasy life does not seem to give you the right degree of excitement, read Nancy Friday's book *Men in Love*. This describes a wide variety of male erotic fantasies and may stimulate your imagination.

☐ Use a vibrator (see below).

Planning your lovemaking

Perhaps the most valuable boost you can give to your lovemaking is to give it enough time, so that it can be as leisurely, sensuous, and prolonged as you like. Plan for it as you would plan for any other worthwhile activity. It is no compliment to your partner, and will almost certainly limit your enjoyment, if sex is usually a last-minute activity, squeezed in after the late movie when you are both almost too tired to stay awake.

VIBRATORS

As a sex aid, vibrators are generally more rewarding for women than for men. They operate at different frequencies, but the most effective frequency is about 80 Hz and, since battery-operated vibrators usually work at a lower frequency, an electric model is probably best. For the most intense sensations, place the head of the vibrator against the highly sensitive underside of the head of your penis – the area known as the frenulum (see p.75).

You can also use the vibrator to stimulate your partner's clitoris directly, and most women can reach orgasm this way, even if they have difficulty doing so during intercourse or through manual stimulation. Some models have a head that is designed to apply particularly intense stimulation to the clitoris and are for use exclusively in this way. Others can be strapped to the back of your hand so that vibrations are transmitted indirectly to the clitoris as you caress it. You can also use this second type of vibrator to give your lover a pleasantly different overall massage. Vibrators will teach you both more about your bodies' responses.

Using a vibrator ▷

The choice of vibrators is extensive. Size does not matter, but the shape of the head is important since it does most of the work in clitoral stimulation. If your partner finds direct contact too intense, apply indirect pressure through the folds of the vaginal lips, or stimulate the vaginal entrance.

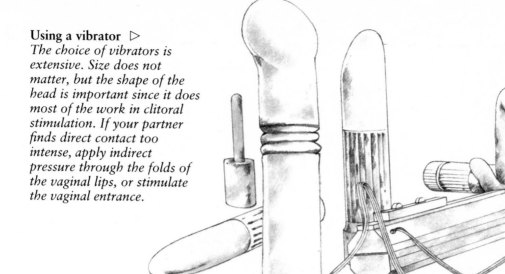

▽ Stimulating the clitoris

The most effective use of a vibrator is in stimulating the clitoris. If your partner finds direct contact too intense, try applying indirect pressure through the folds of the vaginal lips, or (right) using just the head to stimulate the vaginal entrance.

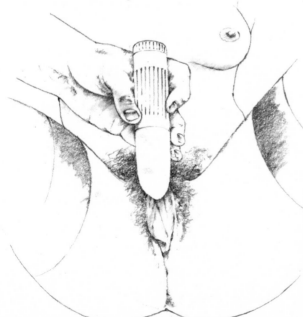

AIDS PRECAUTIONS

To avoid the risk of AIDS, vibrators – and any other sex toys that you use – should never be shared unless they are cleaned thoroughly after use. The HIV virus is destroyed by ordinary household disinfectant or bleach, and also by dish-detergent diluted in hot water.

OVERCOMING INHIBITIONS

Inhibitions are feelings that interfere with your natural sexual response and so prevent you from enjoying sex or even becoming aroused. Nearly always they are the result of experiences that have made you feel guilty or anxious about sex; a puritanical upbringing, for example, or a disastrous episode in adolescence.

Few of us are entirely free from such hang-ups, but they are seldom so severe that they limit our sex lives significantly. Usually we can avoid the particular circumstances or activities that make us feel uncomfortable, but in extreme cases inhibitions may seriously disrupt the whole of your sex life, making you suppress your feelings or even avoid sex completely. The aim of the self-help programs described below is to enable you to modify old attitudes and patterns of behavior or to replace them with new and more flexible ones.

Dealing with sexual guilt

If you feel guilty about sex, you need to give yourself 'permission' to be sexual and to believe that sexual pleasure is something that everyone has a right to. The aim of the following advice is to increase your sexuality, which you may have so consistently and successfully repressed that you think of yourself as someone who has little interest in or desire for sex.

☐ *Develop your fantasy life.* This is a good place to start, because it is safer to let go of your inhibitions in your imagination than in reality. If you find it hard to conjure up fantasies, use sexually explicit magazines or books to stimulate your imagination and examine any long-suppressed sexual feelings. Do not worry if they include people other than your partner; or practices you have no real wish to try: very few people act out their fantasies in reality. However, investigating and elaborating upon fantasy can gradually alter your sexual preference (see p.121), so it may not be a good idea to let your fantasies run totally free.

☐ *Learn to like your body.* The exercises in GETTING IN TOUCH WITH YOUR BODY, p.74, and GIVING YOURSELF PLEASURE, p.77, are an important part of this program. They will help you to feel comfortable with your body and sexual feelings.

☐ *Reassess your attitudes.* Take a fresh look, in the light of adult experience, at the sexual views and attitudes you acquired as a child. Rigorously examine any preconceptions as though you were considering them for the first time. Are they based largely on an emotion that is hard to justify rationally? If so, try to jettison them.

☐ *Become a hedonist.* A common characteristic of men who carry a heavy load of sexual guilt is that they cannot help believing that all pleasure for its own sake is wrong. If you are the kind of person who feels guilty about, say, relaxing instead of working constantly, or about spending money on occasional luxuries, you most likely feel uneasy about enjoying life too much. Make yourself more receptive to pleasure by creating space in your life for sensual enjoyment – of food, music, pictures, or erotic literature, for example. This should make it easier to view sex as another source of legitimate pleasure.

☐ *Learn not to be a spectator.* If you have always had difficulty in accepting your own sexual feelings you probably tend to stand back mentally when you are having sex, disassociating yourself by thinking about other things or watching rather than feeling your own performance. When you have sex, try to concentrate on what you feel, tune in to the sensations you experience, and be aware all the time of your partner's body as you touch her and yours as she touches you. The sensate-focusing exercises in LEARNING TO SHARE PLEASURE, p.79, are one way of practising this concentration on pleasure.

☐ *Letting yourself go.* If you feel inhibited in your sex life, you may be disturbed by the idea of losing control when you make love, of appearing vulnerable, ridiculous, or simply undignified. Maybe you have always made love in silence because it seems to draw less attention to what you are doing, or because you were made to feel as a child that it was somehow animal-like to let go or to show enjoyment. One of the ways to overcome this is to practise a deliberate loss of self-control in sex. For example, respond to your feelings by moving more, breathing more heavily, or yelling, expressing the pleasure you feel in any way you like. You will probably find it easier to do this first when you masturbate.

Dispelling sexual anxiety

Many men think that sexual difficulties begin only in bed and exclusively concern their ability to perform successfully. This 'performance anxiety' is discussed in detail in OVERCOMING ERECTION PROBLEMS, p.87. For a large number of men, though, anxiety about sex is not limited to worries about performance, but extends to their ability to make any kind of close or sexual relationship with women. If you are in this position, use the minimal dating program below to take gradual steps toward a normal social and sexual life. If you have been anxious about sex for so long that you have avoided contact with women for some time, start at the beginning of the program. If you feel comfortable about being on friendly terms with women, but have difficulty turning a social, platonic relationship into a sexual one, start at step 3.

MINIMAL DATING PROGRAM

You will find it easier to use this program if you also read DEVELOPING SOCIAL AND SEXUAL SKILLS, p.146.

1 Your first goal is to make a 'neutral' date that will provoke as little anxiety in you as possible. It should be with a woman you like but not one you find especially attractive. Choose a place or activity without strong romantic overtones: lunch in a popular restaurant, a drink at lunchtime or after work, or a visit to an art gallery or concert, for example. Repeat this undemanding kind of dating a few times until your anxiety has decreased to more manageable proportions.

2 The next step is to make a date with a woman to whom you *are* attracted and, if possible, one who you think might find you attractive. You will feel much more tense about this but, once again, keep the activity neutral and the relationship platonic.

3 Now place your friendship on a more sexual footing. Resolve, though, that you are not yet going to have sex with your date, even if she indicates that she would like to. But you should let her know you are attracted and find out if she feels the same way. You can show as much physical affection as you choose, provided you do not end up in bed. Dine at home by candlelight, or in a frankly romantic restaurant, or choose a sexy movie and hold her hand, in order to step up the sexual pace. You will probably need to push yourself a little, but not so much that you become unbearably anxious again. Some increase in tension is natural if you are (as you should be) genuinely interested in the woman you are with. If you make no progress at all, something is lacking: either courage on your part or the necessary sexual spark between you. If you are holding back because of a fear of rejection, this is the moment to take a few risks. By continuing to try, you increase your chances of success as well as failure.

4 Once you have achieved a little closeness with someone you are attracted to and who seems to feel the same way about you, you will need to confront the underlying problem: anxiety about your sexual performance. There are two very different approaches you can take:

(i) If you feel you know the woman well enough to be to some extent confident of a sympathetic reaction, simply tell her. Explain that you have had problems in the past and, although you very much want her, you are worried they might recur. You may well find that your openness improves your standing with her and allows you to become more trusting of each other. If so, your anxiety will probably decrease. However, if she is unsophisticated, inexperienced, or easily embarrassed, your revelations may make her so uncomfortable that she will be unable to help you. A further difficulty is that for many men the thought of disclosing their problem is even more anxiety-provoking than the problem itself. In both cases the second approach may be better.

(ii) Trust to luck. Go right ahead without preparing your partner for the possibility of failure. There may be no failure, especially if, having made contact with a woman again, you have managed to become slightly less self-critical and anxious about your performance. And even if things do not go as well as you had hoped, you will at least have achieved greater intimacy, which will make it easier for you to talk about your problem.

OVERCOMING THE FEAR OF INTIMACY

Within the framework of a close relationship, sex is safe: you can communicate your needs and show your feelings without fear of rejection or ridicule. But many men, even though they may acknowledge a need for more closeness in their relationships, find it hard to achieve. Indeed, they often fear it and fight shy of it.

If you want to feel closer to your partner, the following suggestions will help. Because you are attempting to change a very fundamental part of your nature you will need a high degree of commitment, but the rewards, in your sexual and your emotional life, will be correspondingly great.

☐ Choose the right partner, or at least minimize your chances of choosing a totally unsuitable one. See MAKING A LASTING RELATIONSHIP, p.144, which shows how you sabotage your own chances of success by becoming involved in a relationship that is very likely to fail.

☐ Set aside some time when you can talk daily to your partner about what has happened to you during the day and discuss problems. Make a special effort to talk about what matters most to you and do not avoid emotional or sexual issues. LEARNING TO COMMUNICATE, p.114, will help you here.

☐ Let your partner see the 'bad' side of you. It is easy to let anyone know the good things about you, but much more difficult to expose aspects of yourself about which you feel worried, guilty or ashamed. However, it is revealing these problem areas that makes for true intimacy.

☐ Show your feelings. Affectionate touching is the most straightforward way of demonstrating a need to be close. Show anger, too, if you feel it, but not in a destructive way. See **Dealing with anger**, p.115.

☐ Give your partner the opportunity to do things for you, letting go of your emotional independence a little. It is particularly important to be able to ask for things sometimes. In doing this you will be acknowledging that you have needs and allowing your partner to meet them.

☐ Spend time together on leisure activities. Do not use excuses such as the pressure of work to avoid spending time alone with your partner.

☐ Do not distance yourself, by provoking a quarrel, for example, whenever you sense that your partner is getting too close to you.

☐ Do not focus on your partner's shortcomings or least attractive features so that you lose sexual interest in her as soon as you feel you are becoming more involved than you want to be.

☐ The sensate-focusing exercises in LEARNING TO SHARE PLEASURE, p.79, are designed to foster intimacy. However, it is important to realize that these exercises provide you with an excellent opportunity for employing all the tactics to avoid intimacy which contribute to your problem. Do not allow yourself to be too tired or too busy to do them, or to remember past injustices and notice physical imperfections as soon as you begin to feel emotional and physical satisfaction.

ANXIETY ABOUT SEXUAL ODORS AND SECRETIONS

If you are bothered by the inevitable smells and messiness of sex, it may be because you have come to associate sex with excretion. The two functions are, in fact, quite separate and if the genitals are kept clean by daily washing they do not normally smell. When you are sexually aroused though, your genitals do have a characteristic odor, and so do your partner's. Most people find this not only pleasant, but exciting. Furthermore, the sexual secretions – vaginal fluid and semen – are harmless, and almost odorless and tasteless too.

If you are uncircumcised, draw your foreskin back when you wash your penis, otherwise a strong-smelling secretion (smegma) can build up under the foreskin. (See **Talking about sex**, p.114.)

IMPROVING YOUR SELF-ESTEEM

To have self-esteem is to feel that you are worth something. A poor self-image affects not only the way you behave toward other people – shyness and jealousy are nearly always the result of low self-esteem, to take prime examples – but also the way they behave toward you, because people tend to accept you at your own self-evaluation. A lack of self-esteem puts you at a disadvantage in social situations, because fear of being rejected usually makes you overeager to please others and very reluctant to risk giving offense. And, naturally, your self-esteem has a direct bearing on your confidence about attracting and retaining sexual partners.

Causes of low self-esteem

Timidity and a sense of the inevitability of failure may be built into a man's personality as the result of an upbringing by parents who were too strict, over-critical, or even unloving. A child will accept his parents' view of him; if they do not make him feel good, lovable and successful, it it not surprising that he grows up believing he is of little worth. Often, too, a man's self-image is colored by childhood teasing that made him believe he was unattractive, or by unsuccessful adolescent experiences of sex that made him feel inadequate.

Even a normally self-confident man may suffer a temporary loss of self-esteem if he fails in an area that is important to him. A setback at work or the break-up of a relationship that means a lot to him will diminish his sexual confidence as well as affecting his general outlook.

Dealing with temporary setbacks

When you have suffered a major blow to your self-esteem it is important first of all to try to see your failure in perspective, as only part of you and your life, not the whole of it. Focus on other areas in which you have had more success. For the time being, concentrate your energies on something at which you are unlikely to fail and which will restore your self-image. For example, after the break-up of an affair, you may find it helps to immerse yourself in your work more than usual, or to start on a new and adventurous project.

Remember that after any loss of prestige or self-esteem, whether at work or in a relationship, you may be tempted to embark on an affair simply because it seems to be the easiest and quickest way to soothe your bruised ego. Such rebound affairs are a risky way to deal with the problem because they are likely to lead to another failure. It is probably better to wait until you have regained your emotional equilibrium.

If, in two or three months, you still feel at a disadvantage sexually, your problem may be more deep-seated. The program that follows is designed to help you overcome such difficulties.

PROGRAM FOR IMPROVING YOUR SELF-ESTEEM

This program, divided into an assessment section and a self-improvement section, will help you to build up your self-esteem and begin to accept yourself as a sexually desirable male. Other parts of the book form essential complements to the program, and you will be directed to these at certain points.

1 ASSESSMENT

Assess your strengths and weaknesses by compiling two lists. First, list your good points, intellectual and emotional as well as physical; secondly, list your faults – the things about yourself that you wish were different or could be improved. Bear in mind the following suggestions:

☐ Try to be specific. Do not simply put down 'good-natured' or 'ugly,' for example. Work out how you are positively good-natured (you like kids, you are a free spender, etc) or negatively ugly (you are pimply, fat, bald, etc).

☐ Do not be tempted to overlook or minimize your strengths. Nearly everyone remembers to write down 'acne' if he has it; far fewer will remember to give themselves credit for a clear skin.

☐ Include among your strong points attributes or skills not directly related to sexual competence. Are you a handyman, for example, or do you play a sport reasonably well? Similarly, if someone else has a talent you admire and believe would give you more self-confidence if you had it – an ability to play the guitar, or skill with computers, for example – list it among your weaknesses.

Now analyze your lists, beginning by comparing them. Are the weaknesses far more numerous than the strengths? If so, why? Perhaps you are being unfair to yourself. A poor self-image may be making you so self-critical that you have dismissed some of your good points as unworthy of mention.

Examine your list of strengths. Are you making good use of those you do have? If there are situations in which you shine, how often do you find yourself in them? If you have a good eye for a ball and enjoy tennis, for example, have you joined a club? Do you even play regularly? And what about your best features? If you are tall, inspect your posture, for a round-shouldered slouch negates the positive aspects of height. If your eyes are one of your most attractive features, learn how to use them to your best advantage. (See **Eye contact**, p.146.)

Finally, examine your list of faults. Delete the ones you can do nothing about. For example, you cannot make yourself six inches taller. The list will still contain a number of things you can change if you are willing to invest time and energy.

2 SELF IMPROVEMENT

The second element of the program will enable you to improve your physical appearance and develop greater self-assurance.

Improving your image
Start with your physical appearance. It is in this area that changes are most easily made and most readily appreciated by others. Would you look better with a different hairstyle or, if you wear spectacles, with contact lenses? Grow a moustache if you think it will suit you; shave off a beard if you suspect it does not.

Look at your clothes. When buying new ones, do not just play safe. Study magazines, advertisements, and store windows, and choose clothes in which you would really feel good. If you have always dressed conservatively, try a more casual approach; if you have been a sloppy dresser, neaten up. Try to buy at stores that suit the image you would like to present. And get good aftershave. This will soon become a pleasantly recognizable part of that image.

Whatever changes you make, introduce them gradually, one at a time, over about six months. This will give you and everyone else time to adjust to them. You will also find it necessary to accustom yourself to other people's changed impression of you. Although this will ultimately boost your self-esteem, it may embarrass you at first if you have always avoided drawing attention to yourself.

Being more confident about your looks
Get to know and like your face and physique as they really are. Too many men feel dissatisfied with their looks not because of gross or obvious abnormalities but simply because they do not add up to their ideal image of a good-looking man. But there is hardly a man who is physically perfect and few women expect physical perfection in their lovers. The exercises in GETTING IN TOUCH WITH YOUR BODY, p.74, should help you gain a more positive view of yourself.

If you have felt sexually inadequate over the size or shape of your genitals, remember that you probably underestimate the size of your penis. The fore-shortened view that you get from above makes it look smaller than it is. Remember, if other men's penises look a lot bigger than yours, that you have probably seen theirs in a resting, flaccid state, and while there is a wide variation in the size of non-erect penises, size differences tend to disappear with erection since small penises swell more than large ones. And remember too that the vagina will mold itself to a penis of any size. The penis you perhaps regard as too small need not lessen your partner's enjoyment, for what you do with it is more important than its size.

Learning to overcome shyness
Over 80 per cent of people questioned in a recent survey said they had felt shy at some time or in some situations, and of these over 40 per cent admitted that shyness was a constant problem for them. So the chances are strong that the person you are too timid to talk to feels much the same as you.

Do not automatically label yourself 'shy'. Instead, regard yourself only as feeling shy in certain situations – in large groups, for example, or with attractive strangers. Giving up the label is the first step toward overcoming the problem itself.

Have faith in your likeability. Shy people usually lack the social skill to make others believe that they are worth knowing. Believe it yourself, and you will communicate your belief without even trying. For this very important part of the program, turn to DEVELOPING SOCIAL AND SEXUAL SKILLS, p.146.

Try not to concentrate on your own feelings of self-consciousness, or to brood about what people think of you. Instead, give your entire attention to anyone you talk to or to any situation, whether sexual or not, that you find yourself in. Some psychologists suggest that an excellent way to overcome shyness is to become involved in a social or political cause. Involvement of this sort provides an opportunity to make a fresh start as an unshy person in a non-sexual situation. A sense of sexual ease should soon follow. You may also find it helpful to read **Dispelling sexual anxiety**, p.69.

It is worth remembering, too, that women are probably less dependent on the physical attractiveness of their partner for arousal than men are. Dress and appearance matter rather less to them (although this does not mean you will be an instant success if you are dirty, scruffy, or unkempt); manner, personality, kindness and consideration count for more.

Finally, make sure you pick the right sexual partner. Many men seem deliberately to sabotage their self-esteem by choosing partners who lower it even more. Not many men can function well with a lover who is critical or rejecting. A partnership based on love and support is essential for anyone whose self-esteem is fragile or for whom self-consciousness is a problem.

Learning to be more assertive

Practise saying no to suggestions you normally, though unwillingly, say yes to. If you have fallen into a pattern of habitually doing something you dislike just because you think it is expected of you – seeing too much of your partner's, or even your own, relatives when you have little in common, for example – break the habit. If your partner regularly pressures you into watching her favorite TV program, invite her to watch yours next time. Assertiveness should not be equated with aggressiveness. It simply means expressing the way you feel and implies no criticism of your partner or others for feeling or wanting something different.

Do not be afraid to ask for things you want. Start by requesting small favors of friends. You might ask if you can borrow something, for example. Or ask someone to pick up the occasional item for you if he or she is going shopping. Sometimes even these small requests will not be granted (other people are assertive too) but part of learning assertiveness is being able to accept an occasional rebuff without interpreting it as a serious rejection.

Practise making decisions and, if they are minor, do not spend time worrying about whether they are right or wrong. A good starting point is to resolve never to say, 'I don't really mind' when you are asked whether you prefer one thing to another. If you have a preference, make it known. Even if you really do not care, make a firm, immediate decision.

Take deliberate risks by acting out of character sometimes. It helps if you can think of it as 'acting'. Allow yourself to seem to lose your temper, for example, if the occasion is right and everyone knows you are a man who never loses his temper. Their impression to date may well be that you do not dare to lose your temper, and their realization that you can show anger, when appropriate, may do wonders for your reputation and consequently for your self-confidence.

Make a deliberate effort to do something you find especially difficult, such as striking up a conversation with strangers or making a justified complaint. Sometimes you may get the snub or even the hostile reaction you dread, but most often you will receive a satisfactory response and a large boost to your self-esteem.

When you have gained confidence and feel more comfortable about asking for what you want among acquaintances and friends, introduce a little more assertiveness into your sexual relationships. You may find this difficult if it involves discussions about sex and your sexual feelings, but LEARNING TO COMMUNICATE, p.114, will help you overcome the problem.

Assessing your progress

After you have worked on the above program for three months, check your progress by answering once again the questionnaire CONFIDENCE, p.16. Compare your result with your previous rating. Has there been any improvement? Check whether your answers pinpoint any specific area you can work on. If your rating is still low, concentrate on **Learning to be more assertive**, above.

Remember that you are trying to change ideas about yourself that you have probably held for most of your life. Do not be discouraged if, like most old habits, they die hard. If you are determined to change and to give up an outdated view of yourself, and if you are willing to take a few risks and expose yourself to a few minor disappointments, you will almost certainly win through.

GETTING IN TOUCH WITH YOUR BODY

The sight and feel of each other's bodies is one of the special joys of lovemaking and, particularly in the early stages of a relationship, a couple can derive almost as much pleasure from exploring each other as from intercourse itself. Naturally, your enjoyment of sex will be diminished, or even prevented altogether, if you are embarrassed about being naked in front of your partner, or if you are at all self-conscious about the way your body looks.

The chemistry of attraction
Self-consciousness usually springs from the belief that you are unattractive on account of physical imperfections. And yet bodily perfection is, as far as the majority of women are concerned, irrelevant to whether or not they find a partner sexually attractive. The chemistry of sexual attraction is so subtle, unpredictable and idiosyncratic that it is often incomprehensible to anyone but those involved.

Your partner's view of you will be quite different from your own or that of anyone else, and she may even find especially endearing the characteristics that you regard as flaws.

Learning to accept your body
The following exercises should help to lessen your self-consciousness, and make you more comfortable with yourself and more aware of your body as a resource for sexual pleasure. The exercises might seem narcissistic at first, and it is quite probable that you will dislike the idea of doing them, especially if, like many men, you seldom use a mirror except to shave or straighten your tie. However, it is important to understand that the aim of the program is not to encourage self-love but to boost self-confidence. In order to feel as relaxed as possible when doing the exercises, you should also ensure that you have privacy and plenty of time.

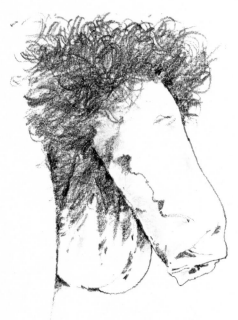

△ **The non-erect penis**
At rest, the penis is about half as long as it is during arousal, when the spongy tissue becomes engorged with blood to produce an erection.

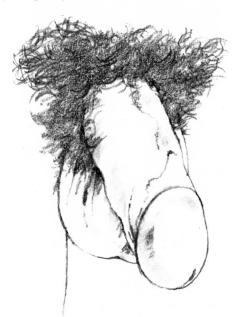

△ **Circumcision**
This surgical operation, which is usually carried out for religious or or medical reasons, removes the foreskin that covers the head of the penis.

1 Study your naked body in a full-length mirror. Look long and hard at your face and then let your eyes travel slowly down to your toes. Imagine that you are seeing yourself for the first time. Look from every angle, and watch yourself kneeling, bending, sitting, moving around. Look over your shoulder to examine your back and the set of your buttocks.

2 Note what is special about you; not perfect, but special. These are the features that make you unique, the qualities that appeal to any woman who finds you sexually attractive.

3 Like everyone else, you have a mix of good and not-so-good features. Look at your body again, but this time focus your attention on your best points. Gloss over the ones you dislike, regarding them as part of the whole, but not a part that matters all that much. They are there, so accept them, but do not dwell on them to the exclusion of everything else.

4 Now study your genitals. Feel your testes. One, usually the left, hangs slightly below the other. This is normal. Look at your penis. When not erect, it is probably between two and four inches long. As you

know, it lengthens considerably when erect. This is because its three cylinders of spongy tissue become engorged with blood when you are sexually aroused. These cylinders are enclosed in a fibrous sheath, and as the spongy tissues fill and press against the sheath, the penis hardens. Let your fingers play on the surface of your penis. You will probably find that the most sensitive area is the head and, in particular, the ridge on the underside where the head joins the shaft. This is known as the frenulum.

5 Finish the exercise by taking a warm bath. Soap your hands and explore your body with them. Notice the different sensations you experience by varying your touch and pressure, and identify the changes in skin sensitivity from area to area. Explore your genitals again too, but do not spend much time on them. The aim of this part of the exercise is to become aware of sensations in the whole body.

6 Dry yourself. Again, focus on sensations and do not be in too much of a hurry.

7 If you like the idea, try using a body lotion and enjoy the feeling as you rub it into your skin.

The frenulum

The head of the penis is more sensitive than the shaft, and the ridge of skin on the underside is particularly well provided with nerve-endings. This is known as the frenulum.

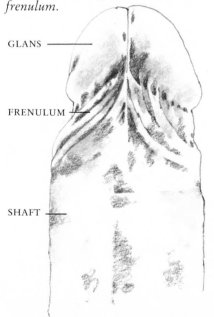

GLANS

FRENULUM

SHAFT

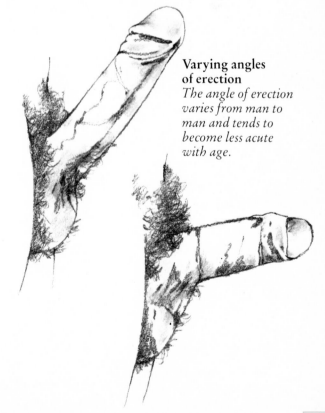

Varying angles of erection

The angle of erection varies from man to man and tends to become less acute with age.

Assessing your progress

By repeating the exercise several times over the course of three or four weeks you can develop a positive image of yourself as you really are, without making adverse comparisons with the body you formerly wished you possessed. Do you feel reasonably comfortable doing the exercise? And do you feel you would now be equally at ease with your sexual partner? If so you can increase your body awareness still more by practising with her the sensate-focusing exercises on p.79.

If, however, you feel you have made little progress it might be helpful to take a different approach. Try a sauna or massage, for example. Both experiences will help you focus your attention on your body as a source of pleasure. Other sections of the book may be helpful too, particularly IMPROVING YOUR SELF-ESTEEM, p.71, and OVERCOMING IN-HIBITIONS, p.68. These are both aimed at helping you feel more relaxed about yourself as a sexually active person, so that you will be more at ease in a sexual relationship.

▽ **Getting to know your body**
The ultimate aim of the preceding self-examination exercises is to feel unself-conscious about your body when with a sexual partner. But first you must become familiar and relaxed with it when alone. Your progress will be faster if you ensure that you have adequate time and complete privacy for the exercises.

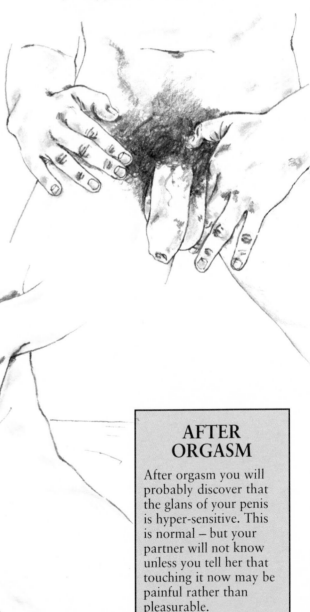

AFTER ORGASM

After orgasm you will probably discover that the glans of your penis is hyper-sensitive. This is normal – but your partner will not know unless you tell her that touching it now may be painful rather than pleasurable.

GIVING YOURSELF PLEASURE

It is not so long ago that the term 'self-abuse' was a popular synonym for masturbation. This attitude began to change rapidly after 1948, when the Kinsey Report (*Sexual Behavior in the Human Male*) revealed not only that over 90 per cent of American men had masturbated, but that its only harmful effect was to give many of them a groundless sense of anxiety and guilt. Modern physicians and psychologists agree that masturbation is a matter of self-pleasuring rather than self-abuse; nor is it regarded simply as a means of relieving sexual tension for the man without a partner, but as an acceptable way for almost every man to learn how best to satisfy his sexual needs.

But even though you may accept rationally that masturbation is both harmless and widely practised, you may still have some reservations about it. It is worthwhile making the effort to overcome these inhibitions, and you will find that the exercise program which follows will help you in this and promote your sexual self-discovery.

Giving yourself maximum pleasure
This program will also help any man who feels reluctant to touch his penis, but prefers to masturbate by rubbing his genitals against something. If you dislike touching your penis you are likely to feel uncomfortable when a woman caresses it, which will make it difficult for you to enjoy sex.

You will want privacy and plenty of time to do these exercises, particularly if you have always regarded masturbation as something to be done furtively and hurriedly. The aim is to discover the sensations that are most pleasurable and to enjoy them in a relaxed, comfortable way. It does not matter if you do not reach orgasm, or even fail to get an erection; you will still have learned much about the kind of stimulation that gives you the most pleasure. You may need some erotic stimulation, books or pictures for example, to arouse fantasies before masturbating.

1 Try to discover which areas of your penis are most sensitive, touching each in turn, and varying the degree of pressure you apply. Whether or not you are circumsized makes no difference to the sensitivity of your penis.

2 If you are uncircumcized, draw the foreskin back and forth over the head until your penis is erect.

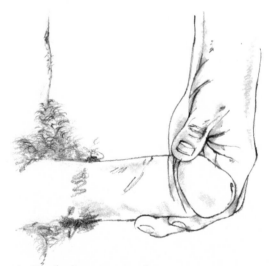

△ **Exploring your penis**
Stimulate your penis by hand in different ways in order to discover which parts, and what kinds of touch, give you the most pleasure.

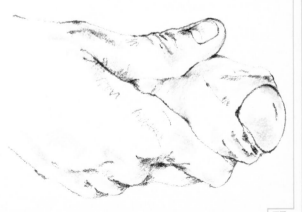

▽ **Sensitivity of the penis**
There is no difference in sensitivity between the exposed head of the circumcized penis and the head of the uncircumsized penis, shown here. In both cases the underside of the head is the area most susceptible to pressure.

Masturbating

When you have a firm erection, start to rub the skin on the shaft up and down, varying the rhythm and the length of the strokes in order to experience as wide a range of sensations as possible.

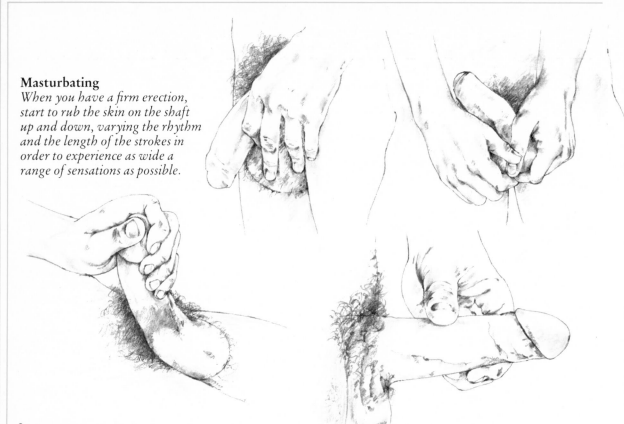

3 If you are circumcized, try alternately squeezing and releasing your penis. You should soon develop an erection.

4 Now stroke the shaft of the penis, varying the pressure you use. Experiment to see whether you prefer a rapid downward movement followed by a slow upward one, or vice versa. Do not rush it.

5 If you feel you are about to reach orgasm before 15 minutes have passed, stop. When the urge to ejaculate has subsided, start stroking again.

6 When you have grown so excited that you can no longer hold back, let yourself go thoroughly, focusing your mind only on the sensations involved.

Assessing your progress

If you enjoy the exercise program and find you can keep going without reaching a climax too soon then you are doing well. If the sensations are less intense than you think they should be, try using a lubricant such as KY jelly or a massage lotion. Often this enhances sensations and makes it easier to focus on them. You can also employ fantasy, or erotic magazines or books, to increase your arousal. If you

find, after doing it a few times, that the exercise still makes you feel very tense, relax for a few minutes beforehand.

ANTICIPATING EJACULATION

Are you unable to stop yourself reaching a rapid climax? If so, you have not yet learned to 'read' the body signals which indicate that ejaculation is inevitable. If this remains a problem after you have been doing the exercise for two to three weeks, you will do best to study DELAYING EJACULATION, p.90.

It is possible that you may find the exercise difficult if you do not normally use your hands to masturbate. If this is the case, masturbate next time in your usual way, but touch your penis just before you ejaculate. From then on, each time you masturbate, stroke and caress it a little earlier each time. Eventually, you will find that you can ejaculate easily by means of manual stimulation.

LEARNING TO SHARE PLEASURE

The following exercises are known as 'sensate focusing' exercises because they help you and your partner focus on the sensations that are produced by exploring each other's bodies. They involve a program of intimate stroking and stimulation that stops short of intercourse.

SENSATE-FOCUSING EXERCISES

Learning to concentrate on your body's sensations can help to freshen any partnership, but it is particularly important for a man who has trouble relaxing and enjoying sex because of qualms about intercourse or physical intimacy in general. Men sometimes fear that something is expected of them by their sexual partner that they may not be able to deliver, and the anxiety that this causes leads to tension. This is why these exercises do *not* involve intercourse (or even, initially, genital contact). Their purpose is to guide you toward enjoyment of physical contact as an end in itself, without the demands of performance. You cannot fail, because you are not being asked to succeed – only to experience. All you need is a willing partner, privacy, and enough time to approach the exercises in an unhurried manner. Both of you should be naked, and many couples find a sensual massage or shared bath helps them relax before starting the exercises.

Regular practice

The exercises are done in a three-stage series. In order to derive the maximum benefit from them, you should try to practise each stage three times a week for two or three weeks before advancing to the next. It is a good idea to make a point of alternating your activities so that the partner who is the first to give pleasure at one session is the first to receive it the next time. Although these exercises are an important part of several self-help therapy programs, any couple can benefit from occasional tender and imaginative sex play in which they try to rediscover all the sensations of which their bodies are capable without setting themselves the usual goals of intercourse and orgasm.

1 PLEASURE IN GIVING

Caressing another person's body is a very special source of pleasure. It need not have any overt sexual content, which is why, during this first stage of the exercises, your attentions do not extend to the genital area. You may find that the pleasure for both of you is increased if the active partner lubricates his or her hands with body lotion.

1 Start the session with your partner lying face down while you kneel either beside or astride her. Gently fondle and stroke her whole body, working your way down from her head to her toes.

2 During this part of the exercise, you are in complete control. Explore your partner's body with your hands and kiss it in any way that feels good to you. She can gently push your hand away if you do something she does not enjoy.

3 After 10 minutes (or longer if you like) change places. Now just relax and enjoy the sensations while your partner caresses and massages you. Feel what is happening to you and focus your attention on each spot she touches. Try not to stand back mentally and watch her.

4 Now you should change position so that your partner can lie on her back while you gently stroke her face and body. (You should avoid touching her breasts or genitals at this stage.)

5 Now lie back while, avoiding your penis and testes, she pleasures you. Do not try to direct or guide her, but if she does something you find uncomfortable, gently move her hand.

6 If you begin to feel at all tense or anxious, ask her to stop for a while but to resume caressing you as soon as you are relaxed again.

7 If you feel sexually aroused at the end of the session, try masturbating. (Your partner should not do this for you at this stage.) However, you might feel so relaxed that you simply fall asleep straight after the session.

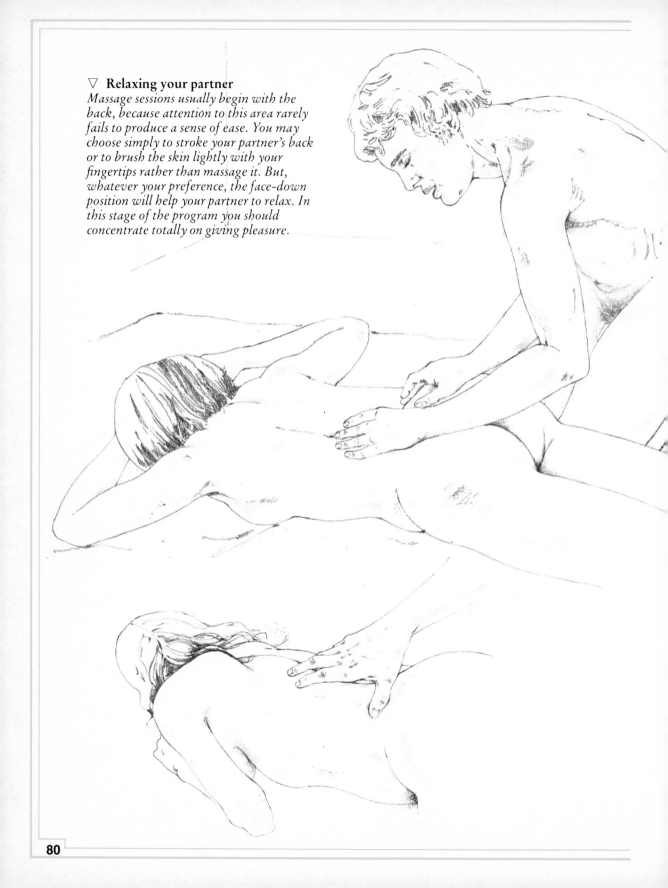

▽ **Relaxing your partner**
Massage sessions usually begin with the back, because attention to this area rarely fails to produce a sense of ease. You may choose simply to stroke your partner's back or to brush the skin lightly with your fingertips rather than massage it. But, whatever your preference, the face-down position will help your partner to relax. In this stage of the program you should concentrate totally on giving pleasure.

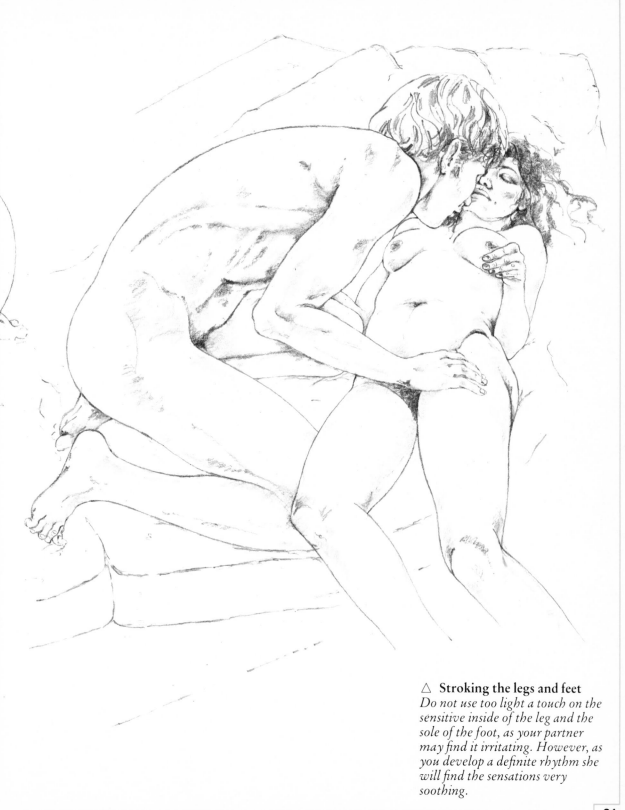

△ **Stroking the legs and feet**
Do not use too light a touch on the sensitive inside of the leg and the sole of the foot, as your partner may find it irritating. However, as you develop a definite rhythm she will find the sensations very soothing.

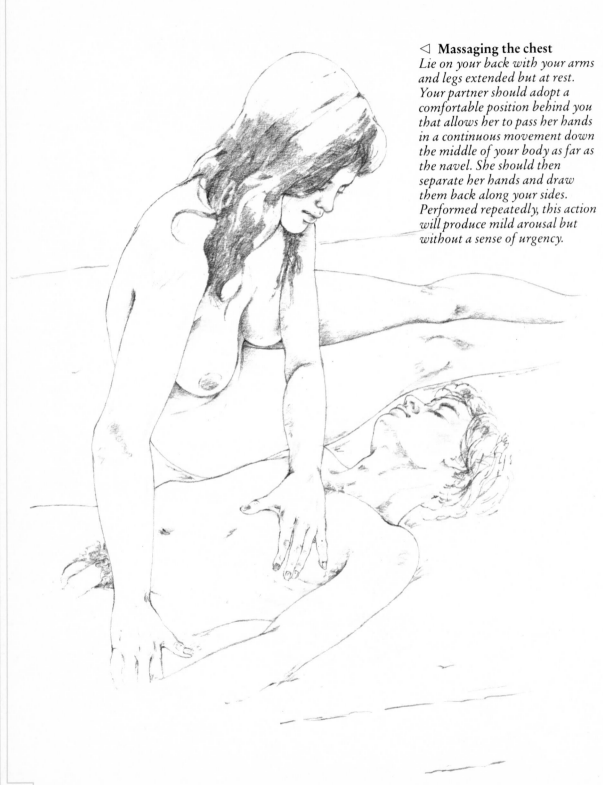

◁ **Massaging the chest**
*Lie on your back with your arms
and legs extended but at rest.
Your partner should adopt a
comfortable position behind you
that allows her to pass her hands
in a continuous movement down
the middle of your body as far as
the navel. She should then
separate her hands and draw
them back along your sides.
Performed repeatedly, this action
will produce mild arousal but
without a sense of urgency.*

Caressing the lower back ▷
To enjoy another very pleasurable
form of caress you lie face down
while your partner sits astride you
and explores the lower part of
your back with her hands.
Concentrate solely on the pleasure
she is giving you and put aside any
feeling of selfishness. If you carry
out the exercises conscientiously,
both of you will learn to give and
enjoy pleasure fully.

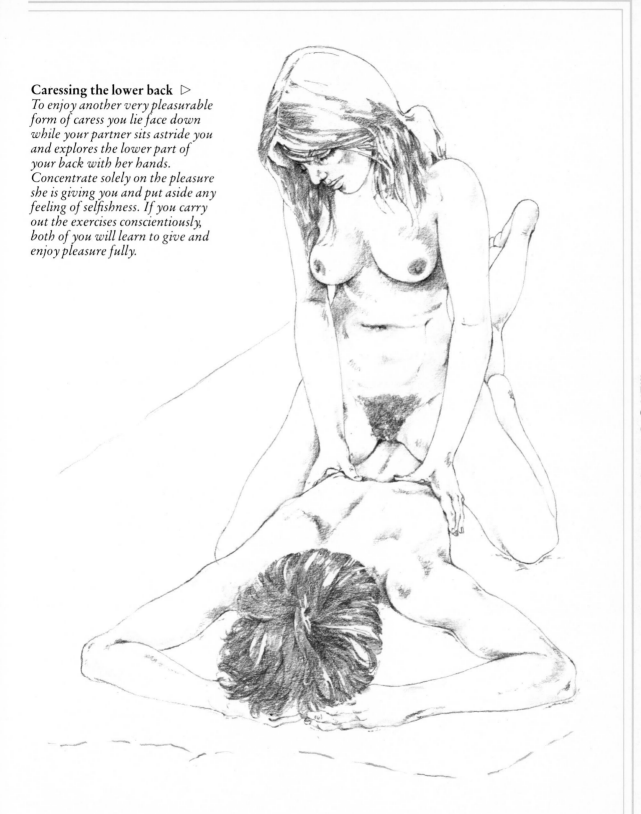

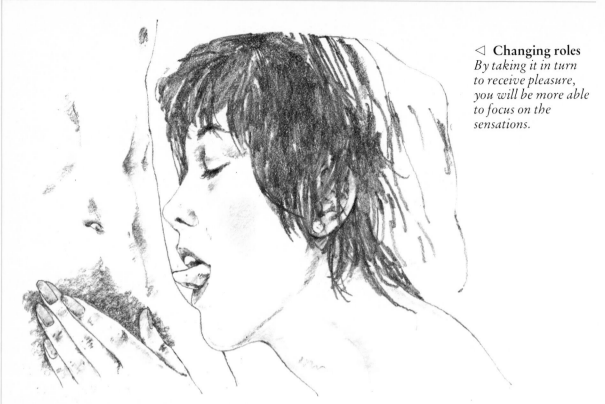

◁ **Changing roles**
By taking it in turn to receive pleasure, you will be more able to focus on the sensations.

2 PLEASURE IN RECEIVING

After practising the preceding exercises for a couple of weeks, move on to the second stage, below. This is a similar set of exercises, except that here the emphasis is on the reactions of the person being caressed rather than on those of the active partner. Instead of simply accepting the attention, the passive partner gives positive feedback to his or her lover about what feels particularly enjoyable. The ban on intercourse and genital touching is still in force.

1 Caress your partner, face-down, then face-up, as before, but try to discover the most sensitive areas of her body and the kind of stimulation she enjoys most. She may, for example, prefer a gentler touch, or perhaps a rougher one, than you yourself would enjoy.

2 Now take your turn, letting her know, in words or gestures, what feels especially good. Guide her hand with yours if you want, and if she kisses you in a certain spot in a way that is highly pleasurable, tell her. Concentrate on your own feelings and do not waste time worrying about whether she might be getting tired or bored. Her turn will come again after 10 minutes or so.

3 At the end of the session, tell each other how you both felt and discuss what most pleased each of you.

Assessing your progress

If, after practising for two to three weeks, you both feel at ease and relaxed with each other during the exercises, you are ready to progress to the third stage. This teaches you how to touch each others' genitals to give maximum pleasure. But do not worry if either of you still feels mildly anxious while doing the exercises. Carry on for another week or so and then, when you feel more comfortable, go on to stage three, which is described below.

Barriers to enjoyment

If you found it was much easier and more enjoyable to caress your partner than to be caressed, it is possible that guilt about sex is inhibiting your enjoyment. Or it may be that you are afraid your partner does not find you attractive, or that the exercise bores her. In each of these cases you cannot concentrate on your own feelings. Try, over the next four sessions, asking your partner for exactly what you want, letting her do only what you ask for. Some men find it easier to lie back and be caressed than to take the active role. If you feel this way, it is worth examining your feelings closely to see whether you have some hostility toward your partner or ambivalence about the relationship which makes it difficult for you to show tenderness and affection. The questionnaires COMPATIBILITY, p.104, and ARE YOU SEXUALLY SATISFIED?, p.109, and the problem chart WHAT IS WRONG WITH YOUR RELATIONSHIP?, p.112, may help you to confront this possibility.

These exercises are designed to promote closeness. If you have encountered within yourself an almost insurmountable resistance to doing them, it is probably because you feel very threatened by the idea of a close relationship. In this case (and likewise if you felt very detached, with no feelings except, perhaps, boredom) you may need professional help to lower your defenses so as to allow yourself to become more emotionally involved.

3 TOUCHING THE GENITALS

You and your partner are now ready to take turns arousing each other by fondling the genitals as well as the rest of the body. Once again, though, stop short of intercourse. The aim of the exercises is simply to fully enjoy this form of contact.

1 With your partner lying on her back, move your hands to her breasts and cup each one so that you can kiss and gently suck the nipples. If your partner is responsive, you will feel the nipples stiffen.

2 Brush your hands across her belly and genital area. Run your fingers through her pubic hair. Be ready to pause for a while if she becomes obviously tense or anxious, but continue these intimate caresses for several minutes.

3 Using a lubricant such as KY jelly, move your fingers lightly around the entrance to the vagina (but not into it) gently stroking it. Then touch the clitoris, which you will feel as a firm spot covered by a hood of skin, at the point where the inner vaginal lips meet at the front. Do not rub hard or use direct pressure, but stroke it softly. The clitoris is a highly sensitive organ with a wealth of nerve endings.

4 Now it is your turn to be fondled. Your partner should stroke your chest and belly, run her fingers through your pubic hair, and caress your inner thighs, moving gradually up to your testes, which she should caress and squeeze gently.

5 Concentrate on your body and the way it responds to her touch. Tell her the sort of pressure you enjoy most, and if you begin to feel tense, ask her to stop for a while. It does not matter whether or not you have an erection. Just experience the pleasure of a tender touch on your genitals.

6 Next, sit down in a comfortable position on the bed. Use a pillow or other support if you like. Your

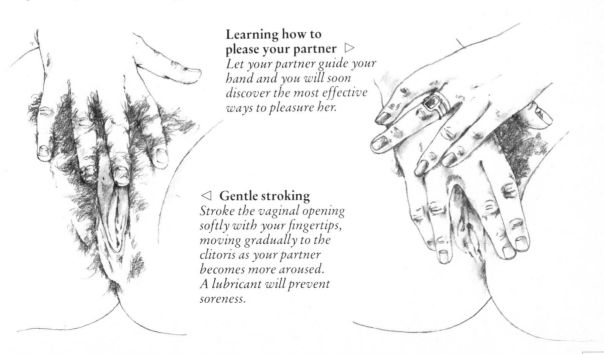

Learning how to please your partner ▷
Let your partner guide your hand and you will soon discover the most effective ways to pleasure her.

◁ **Gentle stroking**
Stroke the vaginal opening softly with your fingertips, moving gradually to the clitoris as your partner becomes more aroused. A lubricant will prevent soreness.

partner should lean back between your thighs, and guide your fingers so that they stimulate her clitoris in the way she likes best. Remember that the clitoris extends much farther than can be seen. Instead of concentrating on the visible tip, you can probably pleasure her most by exerting light pressure on the side of the clitoris through the vaginal lips. Apply saliva or an artificial lubricant and experiment by varying both pressure and tempo. Do not neglect the rest of her body; caress it with your free hand.

7 Change places so that she is sitting and you are lying between her legs. Show her by guiding her hand how to stimulate your penis to produce maximum pleasure, and tell her precisely how you like it. You will almost certainly get an erection, but it does not matter if you do not as you will still feel pleasure.

8 If you have an erection, your partner should play with your penis for a little while, then move her hand to another part of your body and let the erection subside before caressing it again.

9 Orgasm is not the object of this exercise. But if either of you becomes highly aroused you can continue manual stimulation until you climax.

10 Once you both feel quite comfortable doing the exercise you can, if you want, use your lips and tongue to arouse each other (see **Oral sex,** p.52). Your partner will tell you, or push you away gently, if she is not yet ready to try this.

Assessing your progress

If you have both been able to enjoy the preceding exercises without feeling tense or anxious, you can incorporate them into your repertoire of sex play. There will probably be times when, although you do not feel like intercourse, you can enjoy the gentle stimulation of genital pleasuring.

If doing the exercises makes you feel tense or anxious, or if you find yourself switching off by thinking of something quite irrelevant instead of focusing on your feelings, try to relax for a while before starting. Some mild anxiety is natural when you begin to do the exercise. It is possible that you will only feel anxious when it is your turn to be caressed. If so, next time you do the exercise continue to caress your partner, forgoing your own turn. In this way you should gradually become more confident. If you found that you were concerned about genital secretions, odors or appearance – either yours or your partner's – **Anxiety about sexual odors and secretions**, p.70, may be reassuring.

If, after practising the exercises for 4-6 weeks, you have seen no real improvement and still find them difficult, you will probably find professional help valuable (see RESOURCE GUIDE, p.156).

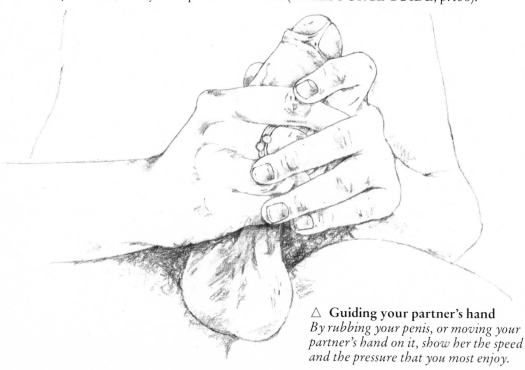

△ **Guiding your partner's hand**
By rubbing your penis, or moving your partner's hand on it, show her the speed and the pressure that you most enjoy.

OVERCOMING ERECTION PROBLEMS

Inability to achieve or maintain an erection is probably the most worrying sexual problem a man can face. The old-fashioned term for the condition – impotence – accurately describes the feelings that such failure produces in a man. In terms of sexual functioning, however, the word is almost useless because it is made to describe every degree of erection failure, from the occasional occurrence, for some trivial reason, to the failure to ever achieve, under any circumstances, an erection.

It is sometimes difficult to decide whether your erectile problems are due to loss of interest in sex (p.24), loss of interest in your partner (p.12), or anxiety about your own failure. Loss of interest in sex in general may be an effect of ageing, but it may also be the result of an illness which your doctor can treat. In this case you will also have lost both the desire to masturbate, and the ability to feel normal sexual attraction.

Difficulty in getting an erection

You may sometimes find you can neither get nor hold an erection, particularly after a heavy drinking session or when you are tired and unenergetic. This is not a serious problem and most men experience such moments. On the other hand, if such episodes have become the rule rather than the exception, consult your doctor as there may be a medical basis for the problem. Similarly, you should see your doctor if you have *never* at any time had an erection: the problem may well have a physical cause.

Physical and hormonal causes of erection problems are quite common, though your anxiety about the problem may intensify it. In some cases there is a pyschological reason for persistent failure. It may be the result of guilt instilled during childhood or adolescence, or it may stem from boredom with a long-standing partnership. Or – and this is probably the most common cause – it can arise because one or two minor episodes become magnified into a major worry about the ability to perform. This 'performance anxiety', inhibits the capacity to achieve and/or maintain an erection.

Occasional erection failure

Almost certainly, at one time or another, you have failed to get an erection when you wanted to, or achieved only a partial erection, or lost it at a critical moment. This can happen if you have sex when you are not really in the mood, or are not fully attracted to the person you are with but have allowed yourself to be drawn into a sexual situation. Sometimes, too, a natural anxiety interferes with your erection. Nervousness in a new relationship or guilt in an illicit one, for example, can do this. Occasional failures of this type are significant only if you immediately label yourself 'impotent'. Using exercise 1 on p. 79, learn to relax before making love so that your erection can develop without your feeling under pressure.

Preventing erection failure

If you find such failures becoming more frequent, it is probably because you expect too much of yourself, or because you are trying to perform under the wrong conditions. The self-help measures suggested below are designed to keep episodes of failure to a minimum. They will help you to avoid the anxiety that can lead to a serious long-term problem.

☐ Have sex only when you are in the mood for it. You are a man, not a machine, and your feelings and your sexual performance will not always be the same. You feel more turned-on at some times than at others, and occasionally you will need extra stimulation. If you have a steady partner, she may not realize this unless you tell her.

☐ Avoid casual encounters – at least until your sexual confidence improves. You will be less anxious with a partner you know and trust.

☐ Do not judge your performance in terms of your penis. Mutual satisfaction is often achievable without intercourse.

☐ If you fail to get an erection, or lose it just before or during intercourse, do not overreact. Simply explain what has happened: 'I guess I'm too tired (I've drunk too much) tonight. Let's try again tomorrow', and do not feel guilty. But do reassure your partner that it is not her fault. Most important, do not withdraw physically or mentally. Stay intimate with your partner in any way you like that does not involve intercourse. If you enjoy being together, erection or not, you will be less anxious about failing next time.

TREATMENT FOR ERECTION PROBLEMS

If erection failure occurs so often that it severely affects your sex life, first consider whether there may be a physical cause. This is more likely if you are older and experienced, and if failure occurs in all situations including masturbation, on waking, and situations where you do not have to perform, such as watching erotic films. The problem may be helped by very erotic lovemaking. In these circumstances, seek your doctor's advice. Otherwise, try the following exercises. Their aim is to dispel your anxiety by helping you accept the fact that even if an erection subsides, gentle stimulation can usually bring it back. In doing these exercises you will be free from worries about your sexual performance because you are not required – in fact, you are not allowed – to have intercourse until you feel confident enough.

The first stage of the exercise can be practised without a partner. Thereafter, though, you need the cooperation of a sympathetic woman who is fond enough of you to undertake with patience and, ideally, pleasure, the gradual steps that comprise the treatment. If you lack a partner at the moment, or if anxiety about 'impotence' has made you avoid relationships, the **Minimal dating programme**, p.69, may help you establish a relationship.

Try to do the following exercises at a time when you feel most in the mood for sex.

1 Begin to stimulate your penis by hand, using whatever fantasy most arouses you, until it is fully erect. (If you cannot get an erection in this way, simply repeat the procedure each day until it works.) Now stop the stimulation and let the erection subside completely. Switching your concentration to some non-sexual subject will hasten this.

2 When your penis is soft, begin to masturbate once more, and when you have a full erection, deliberately lose it again. Then stimulate yourself a third time and carry on until you ejaculate if you feel like it. If you find it difficult to regain an erection after deliberately losing it (or if you cannot get one at the beginning of the exercise) you will find that a lubricant will enhance the sensations considerably.

Repeat this exercise until you are confident that, in solitude at least, you can achieve an erection, lose it voluntarily, and regain it. Confidence should come after the third or fourth repetition of the exercise. You now need a cooperative partner, with whom you should read through the next stage of the program and discuss it. It is important for you both to realize that you have to be selfish, and put your own needs first, if the treatment is to be effective. Your partner must be prepared for some frustration because at this stage you cannot have full intercourse, even though you may both be highly excited. But you can, of course, give her an orgasm either manually or orally at the end of each session.

1 Do together the exercises described in LEARNING TO SHARE PLEASURE, p.79. Simply relax and enjoy being caressed by your partner. Do not worry about whether or not you get an erection.

2 Now your partner tries to stimulate you manually to erection, but not to orgasm. A lubricant enhances the sensations, making it easier to gain an erection.

3 When you have achieved an erection, your partner stops, letting it die away completely, and then begins to stimulate you again. If she is willing to stimulate you orally, you will find this an infallible way of regaining an erection (or of gaining one at the beginning of the exercise if it proves difficult). This step will reassure you that although an erection is lost it can be regained at will. Once you are confident that you can gain, lose, and regain an erection in your partner's presence, have her bring you to orgasm.

Practise these exercises three or four times a week for three or four weeks before you progress to the next stage, below, in which you will learn to relax while in your partner's vagina.

1 Sitting astride you, but without attempting penetration, your partner caresses your penis until you have a full erection.

2 Your partner now guides your penis into her vagina. Concentrate on how this feels for a few moments, and then ask her to move gently. You can thrust if you like, but if you feel you are reaching orgasm, ask her to withdraw from you. Do not ejaculate inside her at this stage. If you lose your erection through anxiety, do not attempt full penetration next time you do the exercise, but just rub your penis between your partner's vaginal lips.

3 When you feel comfortable about vaginal containment, thrust more vigorously, setting a pace that feels right for you. Your partner can increase

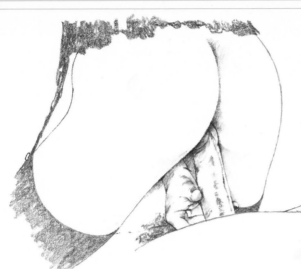

◁ Producing an erection
Having adopted an astride position that is comfortable for both of you, your partner should then caress your penis until it is fully erect.

▽ Enjoying vaginal containment
When your partner has guided your penis into her, concentrate on the feeling of being contained before beginning to thrust.

▽ Caressing the testes
As you develop a rhythm of thrusting, your partner can increase your excitement by reaching down and fondling your testes.

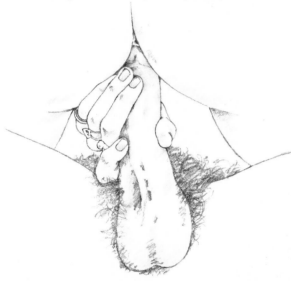

your arousal by stroking your testes or by using her vaginal muscles to squeeze your penis and, if necessary, you can withdraw so that she can stimulate you manually. Withdraw if you feel at all anxious.

4 If you find it hard to ejaculate with your partner on top, adopt a man-on-top position. As your confidence grows, experiment with new positions, but always slow down and simply enjoy being contained if you feel you are losing your erection. (An erection that improves with thrusting but subsides when you slow down, is more typical of a physical problem.)

Assessing your progress
Provided you take the program one step at a time, without feeling you must hurry on to the next stage before you are ready, your sexual performance should become far more reliable within a few months. There may still be times – in a new sexual relationship, for example – when you will feel anxious. But you will have no reason to think of yourself as even slightly 'impotent'. To prevent a real problem from developing again, however, follow the guidelines suggested in **Preventing erection failure**, p.87, in all future sexual encounters.

DELAYING EJACULATION

Ejaculation is a reflex muscular contraction and there comes a point in a man's sexual arousal when it is inevitable. Many men worry because they feel that they reach this point too soon. They often imagine that they and their partner would enjoy intercourse much more, and it would be much easier for the woman to reach orgasm, if they could only hold off ejaculation for just a few minutes longer than normal.

There is, however, no absolute criterion for how long you should last. It is possible that you have unrealistic expectations, so, before deciding you have a 'problem' needing treatment by the 'stop-start' or 'squeeze' techniques described below, try the following approach.

Learning to last longer

Make sure your partner is fully aroused before you start to have intercourse. Foreplay should last 20 minutes at least, so that even if intercourse is brief, lovemaking is not. When you do start to have intercourse, try at first making movements less stimulating than thrusting; a circular movement of the hips to move the penis in the vagina, for example. An even simpler method is to wait 15-30 minutes after you have ejaculated and then, if you can regain an erection, have intercourse again. This time the edge will be off your arousal, so you will probably be able to last longer. This method is especially effective if you are young and sexually inexperienced (as you grow older you will automatically develop a degree of control). Some beginners find that increasing the frequency of masturbation also reduces their sexual tension and enables them to delay ejaculation during intercourse.

However, there are a few men who suffer from a 'hair-trigger' problem: some can manage to thrust a little but still feel they have virtually no control over when they reach a climax, while others ejaculate before they even touch their partner. If you fit into either of these categories, the exercises described here will probably be very successful in helping you to develop greater control.

THE STOP-START TECHNIQUE

The following series of exercises, which was originally developed by Dr James Semans, is aimed at teaching you how to hold your level of arousal just below the point at which ejaculation is inevitable. You do this by gradually learning to recognize the physical sensations leading up to your climax and by modifying accordingly the movements you make during intercourse. Semans discovered that the stop-start technique is of enormous assistance to many of the large number of men who ejaculate so quickly that sex tends to prove disappointing to both themselves and their partners.

Most men who practise these exercises gain good control in 2-10 weeks. You may find, however, that a somewhat different approach, using the 'squeeze' technique developed by Masters and Johnson (see p.93) is more effective for you. In either case you will need the cooperation of a sympathetic partner. Single men, whether heterosexual or homosexual, will find they can gain a good measure of control by practising just the first three steps of the stop-start method. These involve only manual stimulation and do not require the assistance of another person.

1 Masturbate with a dry hand, focusing your attention only on the pleasurable sensations you experience in your penis, not on the sexual fantasies normally associated with masturbation. When you feel you are about to ejaculate, stop and relax. Start again when you no longer feel close to orgasm. Repeat the stop-start procedure, making a conscious effort to stave off an ejaculation, for fully 15 minutes. You may not succeed at first, but continue this preliminary exercise until you have had three consecutive 15-minute sessions without premature ejaculation. The first few times you do the exercise, you will probably have to stop and start quite often, but you will gradually learn to read your body signals more accurately and will need to pause less frequently.

2 The next step is to do the same exercise using a lubricant such as KY jelly. Because this produces much more intense sensations, the timing of your orgasm will be more difficult to control. Again your goal should be to delay ejaculation during three consecutive 15-minute sessions.

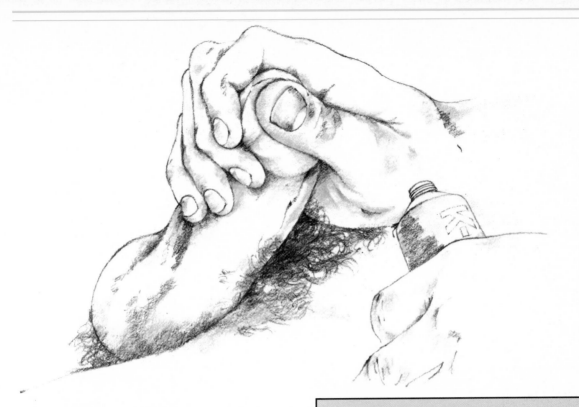

△ **Heightening the sensations**
When you have gained ejaculatory control during masturbation with a dry hand, try to delay orgasm while using a lubricant, which intensifies the sensations. Your excitement will be greater but the stop-start routine will make it possible.

EJACULATORY CONTROL

Do not try to gain increased control either by 'switching off' sexually (thinking about something else during intercourse) or by using ointments that claim to make the penis less sensitive. It is better to gain control by learning to recognize the sensations that build up to orgasm than by trying to ignore or suppress them.

3 You have now developed enough control to try to keep down your arousal without stopping stroking your penis. Masturbate with a dry hand, but whenever you become very excited alter the strokes so that the excitement is eased. To do this, you can either slow down the tempo, use a different type of stroke or degree of pressure, or concentrate on less sensitive areas of the penis. Do not stop altogether, as you did in steps 1 and 2. Experiment in order to find out which method works best for you. The aim is to last 15 minutes – at this stage without stopping – for three consecutive sessions.

4 At this point your partner becomes involved. First, explain to her the procedure you have gone through.

Then ask her to stimulate your penis with a dry hand while you lie back with your eyes closed and concentrate, as you did in the first step of the exercises, on the sensations. As soon as you feel ejaculation is imminent, ask her to stop for a few moments to let the arousal subside. As before, try to last for 15 minutes before ejaculating and take the next step only after three successful sessions.

5 Repeat step 4, but this time with a lubricant. You will find this extremely exciting. Just enjoy the feelings of mounting excitement and let nothing distract you. If you feel close to orgasm too soon, however, ask your partner to stop until the excitement dies down.

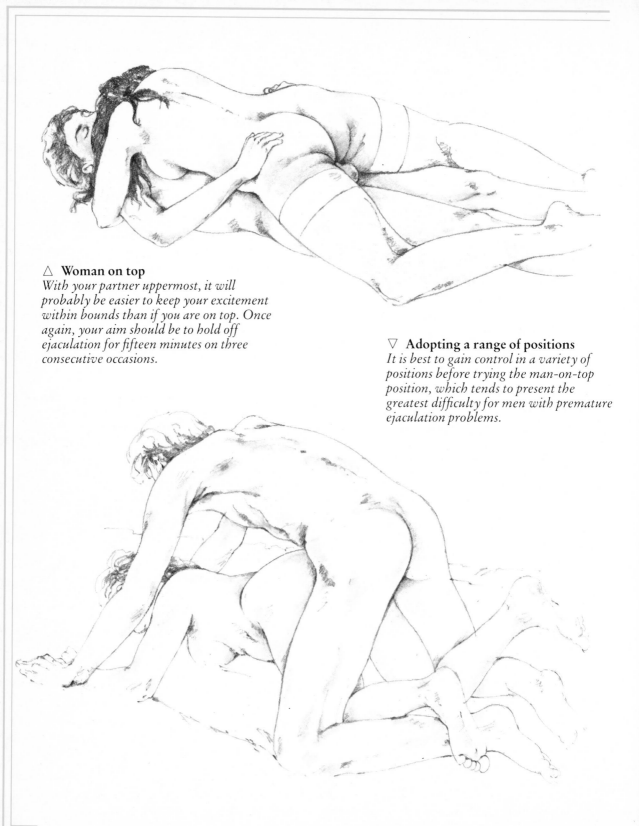

△ **Woman on top**
With your partner uppermost, it will probably be easier to keep your excitement within bounds than if you are on top. Once again, your aim should be to hold off ejaculation for fifteen minutes on three consecutive occasions.

▽ **Adopting a range of positions**
It is best to gain control in a variety of positions before trying the man-on-top position, which tends to present the greatest difficulty for men with premature ejaculation problems.

6 Three consecutive successes in step 5 indicate that you now have enough control to try the stop-start technique during intercourse. The best position at first is with your partner lying comfortably on top of you (see SEXUAL POSITIONS, p.55). When your penis has been inserted, put your hands on her hips to guide her and ask her to move gently up and down. Stop her as soon as you feel you are about to ejaculate, and start again when the urge has gone. Do not thrust; just feel the movement and concentrate on the sensations. Try to last 15 minutes before thrusting and ejaculating. Repeat this type of relaxed intercourse three or four times, permitting yourself each time to thrust more often and more actively, but always stopping if you approach orgasm before the end of 15 minutes. If you ejaculate too soon do not regard this as the end of the exercise: simply relax for at least 15 minutes and then begin intercourse again.

7 Practice intercourse in different positions such as side-by-side or rear-entry before you finally move to the man-on-top position, which is the one in which delaying ejaculation is most difficult.

Assessing your progress

If, after practising the stop-start exercises for at least five weeks, your control is no better, try changing to the squeeze technique described below. Some men find this exercise more effective, but problems sometimes arise because it can seem boring, or because your partner feels frustrated or neglected. However, it is essential for you to concentrate on your own feelings during this period. And because it is an exercise that usually produces good results, the eventual improvement in your sex life should make temporary boredom worth enduring. Your partner need not be frustrated at the end of the session, since after ejaculation you can bring her to orgasm (see STIMULATION TECHNIQUES, p.50). If you have tried both the stop-start and squeeze techniques without success your doctor may be able to prescribe a drug to help you regain control.

It is possible, if it worries you unduly to have to rely on your partner's help during these exercises, that you feel insecure, either about yourself or your relationship. It will help to talk things over with her (see LEARNING TO COMMUNICATE, p.114).

THE SQUEEZE TECHNIQUE

This is a somewhat more complex technique than the stop-start method for treating premature ejaculation. It requires your partner to squeeze your penis in a way that inhibits ejaculation when you feel it is imminent. Let her grip it firmly, using two fingers and the thumb of one hand. Her thumb should be placed on the frenulum, which is the area on the underside of the penis where the head and the shaft meet. Her first finger should be opposite the thumb and the others around the shaft. She should apply fairly firm pressure, without moving her fingers, since too light a touch can arouse you instead of inhibiting ejaculation.

1 Your partner masturbates you as in steps 4 (dry hand) and 5 (with lubrication) of the stop-start technique. But instead of removing her hand when you signal to her that you are about to ejaculate, she squeezes your penis for 15-20 seconds, which causes your erection to subside. She then begins to stimulate you again. Repeat the procedure two to three times before allowing ejaculation to occur.

2 When you have gained a degree of control in this way, you are ready for intercourse; but of a particular kind. Your partner sits astride you and guides your erect penis into her vagina, where it remains with neither of you moving until you warn her (in good time) that you are near orgasm. She immediately lifts herself gently away and applies the squeeze grip. Repeat the exercise two or three times before you let yourself climax.

3 When you are quite sure that your control has improved (this will probably be after you have practised step 2 three or four times) you should try gentle movement during intercourse. Using the same woman-on-top position, begin to thrust a little, and encourage your partner to move her hips slightly. But she should be prepared to withdraw and squeeze whenever you give her the signal. Within a few weeks you should be able to maintain this pause-and-squeeze kind of intercourse for 15-20 minutes without ejaculating.

4 Now attempt intercourse in other positions. You may find that control remains difficult in the traditional male-on-top position. But if you practise step 1 of the squeeze technique at least once a week for the next three months, you should, by the end of that period, have gained ejaculatory control that will be useful in all types of sexual activity.

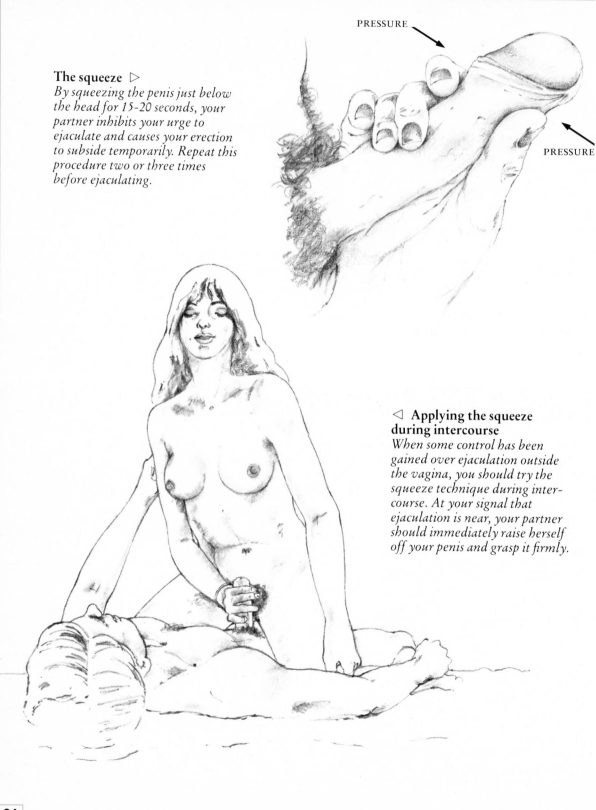

The squeeze ▷
By squeezing the penis just below the head for 15-20 seconds, your partner inhibits your urge to ejaculate and causes your erection to subside temporarily. Repeat this procedure two or three times before ejaculating.

PRESSURE

PRESSURE

◁ **Applying the squeeze during intercourse**
When some control has been gained over ejaculation outside the vagina, you should try the squeeze technique during inter-course. At your signal that ejaculation is near, your partner should immediately raise herself off your penis and grasp it firmly.

SPEEDING EJACULATION

Most men have a degree of control over when they ejaculate. They learn, through practice, how to hold their excitement below the critical level at which orgasm occurs, delaying it until they feel completely ready to let go and climax.

The problem of overcontrol

However, a few men tend to have too much control. Although they feel sexually aroused and have firm erections, they cannot 'let go', so that the normal ejaculatory reflex is inhibited. Anxiety about sex caused by a rigorous religious upbringing, or fear of making your partner pregnant, may contribute to the problem. Often, men with this difficulty tend to be 'super-controlled' people who have difficulty in expressing any strong emotions, or in feeling emotional closeness. Some men may have unwittingly 'conditioned' themselves to ejaculate only when they masturbate.

Sometimes there is a physical basis for the problem: a few drugs inhibit ejaculation (see **The sexual side-effects of drugs**, p.152) and similarly, some medical and surgical conditions (see SEX AND HEALTH, p.151). See your doctor and tell him about the problem if it has developed only recently.

As you grow older, you may need stronger stimulation before you ejaculate, and may not always reach a climax. The ability to last is one of the advantages of advancing age. However, you may need to accept that intercourse will not always end in ejaculation.

True ejaculatory overcontrol may be so severe that the man cannot ejaculate at all, even when he masturbates. This rare problem will almost certainly need the help of a professional sex therapist. The chances are that you have the problem to a much milder degree: perhaps you can ejaculate if your partner stimulates you by hand, but you cannot climax in her vagina, for example.

TREATMENT PROGRAM FOR SPEEDING EJACULATION

The aim of the exercises that follow is to give you intense physical stimulation with progressively closer contact with your partner, but at the same time to distract you so that you cannot easily hold back and exercise too much control over ejaculation. Practise each step of the treatment as often as is necessary to gain complete confidence, and at every stage use fantasy or the memory of past sexual pleasure to increase your excitement.

You may find the first two or three steps of the program easy, but work through them all quickly until you reach your 'sticking point'. Your partner's help will be an essential part of the treatment, so it is important for her to read through the exercises with you so that she understands what she has to do.

1 The first step is to ejaculate comfortably in your partner's presence. Sit close together but with your backs to each other. Masturbate until you ejaculate, using KY jelly or another lubricant. Repeat this step several times until you feel at ease doing it.

2 Now involve your partner. Hold her against you as you masturbate. Practise as often as you need to until you can ejaculate easily while she watches you.

3 Your partner now helps you ejaculate, using manual or – if you both prefer – oral stimulation. Guide her hand to show her the vigorous stimulation you need. She should use plenty of lubricant.

4 At your next session, start to learn to ejaculate progressively closer to your partner's vagina, though not yet inside. She should try to use less vigorous stimulation now, to prepare you for the gentler sensations of vaginal containment.

5 When you are confident you can ejaculate with your partner stimulating you, you are ready to progress to intercourse with ejaculation. Your partner stimulates you until you are close to ejaculation and then you enter her, adopting a position in which she can reach your penis and continue to stimulate it with her hand as you thrust. Ask her to stop when your orgasm is imminent so that you ejaculate through thrusting alone.

6 The final step is to climax through intercourse alone, without additional manual stimulation. However, your partner should stimulate you by hand first, so that you are highly aroused before you

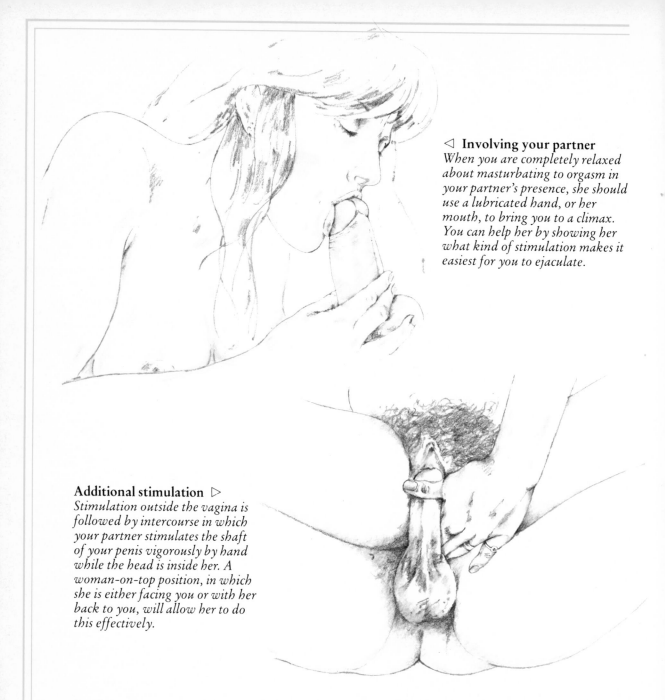

◁ Involving your partner
When you are completely relaxed about masturbating to orgasm in your partner's presence, she should use a lubricated hand, or her mouth, to bring you to a climax. You can help her by showing her what kind of stimulation makes it easiest for you to ejaculate.

Additional stimulation ▷
Stimulation outside the vagina is followed by intercourse in which your partner stimulates the shaft of your penis vigorously by hand while the head is inside her. A woman-on-top position, in which she is either facing you or with her back to you, will allow her to do this effectively.

enter her. A man-on-top position in which her legs are closed is particularly effective because it increases the friction on the penis.

Assessing your progress

If you find that you 'block' at any stage of this program so that further progress seems impossible, it is probable that for some reason you are 'holding back' mentally as well as physically from your

partner. The most common reason for this is a fear of close involvement with women, although there may be a particular conflict in your relationship which needs to be resolved before self-help therapy can be effective. Also, see OVERCOMING THE FEAR OF INTIMACY, p.70, and the problem charts in the fifth part, THE SINGLE MAN, which examine some of the difficulties involved in forming and sustaining relationships.

COMING TO TERMS WITH HOMOSEXUALITY

Life for the sexual minorities has always been difficult, as it has for most minorities. Homosexual men may find that the life they lead is at odds with the life their family and friends believe they are leading. They may want to 'come out', though they are apprehensive about other people's reactions. They may find it hard to accept the fact of their own sexual orientation, or even wish they could modify their sexual preferences to conform with other people's expectations.

Many of the problems gays have arise from the social discrimination, based on prejudice, against them. Sadly, the public's present awareness of the dangers of AIDS, often coupled with a lack of factual knowledge about the disease, has meant that gays are facing yet another rising tide of intolerance. They also have to deal with their own fears about the disease (see **Testing for AIDS**, p.155), and perhaps modify their sex lives to minimize the risks they run with regard to the virus.

Making the choice

The heterosexual male seldom questions his sexual preferences and he is fortunate in that his inclinations fit in with what is expected of him. But if you suspect that your sexual preference is for other men, you are likely to question your own feelings, or sometimes even to go through the motions of a normal heterosexual life, before you can accept that preference. The questionnaire ORIENTATION, p.19, should help you decide where your true inclinations lie, but if you still find it hard to decide, consider the following points:

☐ If you are under 21, do not assume, because you have had some homosexual feelings or experiences, that these have necessarily set the pattern for your adult life. Most men have homosexual encounters at some time in their lives, usually in adolescence. As you have more opportunity to meet women and gain more confidence with them you will probably find that you grow more attracted to them.

☐ You may need to try out a variety of relationships with people of both sexes to discover what suits you best. Do not let yourself be pressured by either gay or straight friends into committing yourself one way or the other until you are really sure about what you really want.

☐ What matters most in deciding on your sexual preference is what arouses you. If you have no sexual interest at all in women, or if you have a strong aversion to heterosexual activity, the situation will not change. However intellectually appealing, however much simpler a heterosexual life might seem, you will do better to accept your homosexual orientation.

☐ If you continue to be troubled by uncertainty about your inclinations, or if you have difficulty in accepting the fact that you are gay, ask your doctor to refer you to a counselor or clinical psychologist.

If there is a quite definite heterosexual element in your make-up (your rating for ORIENTATION will be C-E) you may be able, if you wish, to strengthen the heterosexual side of your personality (see p.98). A homosexual life is not an easy one, and about 20 per cent of gay men marry in an attempt to conceal their true orientation, to deny it to themselves, or to rid themselves of their homosexual impulses. But such relationships are usually troubled and short-lived unless they are based on a core of genuine heterosexual feeling. If women do not arouse you at all, your best policy is to try to accept the fact and adopt a homosexual way of life rather than make yourself and a woman unhappy.

The problems of being gay

If you are homosexual you will encounter the same sexual problems (erection difficulties or premature ejaculation, for example) as other men, but there are a few which are of special concern to gay men. Foremost among these are the social problems of deciding whether, and to what extent, to 'come out'. Probably more than half of all homosexuals decide to tell their families, though no more than a third tell their employers, fellow-workers or friends.

Coming out can obviously make life easier in that there is no longer a need for secrecy or concealment, and yet more difficult in that it may restrict your job options and incur the disapproval of family or friends. This is a decision only you can make, but the chances are that if you do decide to tell the people who matter most to you, they will understand and you will feel, eventually, much more at ease both with yourself and them.

Whether or not you decide to come out completely, you will find it very helpful to have the support of a gay organization through which you can meet homosexual friends. (See RESOURCE GUIDE, p.156). Once you have adopted a homosexual lifestyle, you may feel less need to conceal it from those close to you. Even so, you do not have to make any statements about it if you do not want to.

Sexually transmitted diseases

If you are homosexual you are more likely to catch a sexually transmitted disease (STD) and, in particular, your chances of contracting AIDS (Acquired Immune Deficiency Syndrome) are higher than those of heterosexual men (see SEXUALLY TRANS-MITTED DISEASES, p.153). Single homosexual men are not necessarily more promiscuous than single heterosexual men, but the homosexual lifestyle usually provides partners more readily and so there is a greater risk of infection. The straight male's sexual ambitions are curtailed to some extent by the more monogamous attitude of women. Because of the danger of AIDS and other STDs, many gay men are reducing the number of their sexual partners, and opting for 'safer sex' activities (see **Guidelines for safer sex**, p.154).

The search for a stable relationship

The happiest homosexuals are the ones who have a steady partner and draw most of their emotional and sexual satisfaction from that person. The evidence suggests that gay men are just as dependent for their happiness as heterosexuals on having a close, loving and stable relationship.

Unfortunately, though, homosexual affairs tend to be more numerous, casual, and fleeting than heterosexual ones. Because men usually understand each other's need for sexual variety, such opportunistic liaisons seldom break up a good relationship. But the more casual partners a man has, the more chance there is that one such meeting may develop into a serious relationship. When this happens, the stability of the homosexual couple is just as vulnerable as that of a heterosexual pair.

How to safeguard your relationship

Many gay men do manage, in spite of the difficulties, to make strong and lasting commitments to each other, and, being of the same sex, they are often more companionable and sympathetic to each other's needs and interests than many mixed-sex couples. What can *you* do if you want to increase your chances of a lasting relationship? Here are some tips:

☐ Choose your partner for the right reasons, so that you have more in common than just sex. The advice that is given in MAKING A LASTING RELATIONSHIP, p.144, applies to anyone, whatever their sexual orientation, who is looking for security.

☐ Decide how 'open' you want your relationship to be. However much freedom you intend to give each other, in practice it will work better if you establish certain rules. For example, you may feel more able to take a partner's infidelity if he tells you exactly what is going on, or on the other hand, you may prefer to know absolutely nothing about it. You may agree that there will be no sex with friends and that you will never give your telephone number to casual partners. You may also promise that you will not abandon the other at a party so that he has to come home alone or that, whatever happens, you will always spend the night together.

☐ Stay away from the unattached gay scene as much as you can. Spend your leisure time together and base your social life as much as possible on home and mutual friends, gay or straight.

☐ Remember that the quality of a relationship does not depend on the gender of the people involved. If your relationship is not bringing you much happiness, turn to COMPATIBILITY, p.104. This questionnaire may be used, with appropriate modification, by any gay couple who want to analyze the reasons for their dissatisfaction.

☐ Try to feel positive about your homosexuality. If you see it as wrong, you will find it hard to make good relationships and, at worst, you may tend to sabotage them because you believe you do not deserve to be happy.

Strengthening your heterosexual side

You may, however, want to develop the heterosexual side of your personality but feel that it is impossible to make a successful straight relationship unless you overcome your homosexual feelings altogether. This is not necessarily true, and anyway it is unlikely that your gay inclinations will vanish altogether. But you may be able to make them less important to you. If you can do this, there is no reason why they should threaten a heterosexual relationship. It may help you to consider that while a completely heterosexual man is likely to occasionally fancy women other than his partner, he does not necessarily act on his desires. The following advice will also help you reinforce your heterosexual inclinations.

☐ Masturbate using heterosexual fantasies to heighten your responsiveness to women. At first you may need to keep yourself at a distance in your fantasy, perhaps by simply being an onlooker – imagining another man making love to a woman, for example. You may find yourself concentrating on the man at first, but gradually shape the fantasy so that you pay more attention to the woman, until finally you yourself are playing the male role in your imagination. Monitor your reaction to your fantasies. They should show you what most easily arouses you, and they may help you to focus on any specific

fears you have about heterosexuality – anxiety about being rejected, for example, or an aversion that you have to female genitals. You may find **Sexual phobias**, p.27, helpful if you have the latter problem.

☐ If you have difficulty becoming aroused in your first sexual encounters with women, fantasize about men for the time being.

☐ When you start to (re)discover heterosexual relationships, do not be discouraged if you have some failures. It is important not to give up or to imagine that if you do not succeed immediately you have set yourself an impossible target. Give yourself time and remember that if you do not manage to strengthen your heterosexual side so much that you could fully commit yourself to a woman, you still have your homosexual feelings on which to base relationships. You are therefore losing nothing.

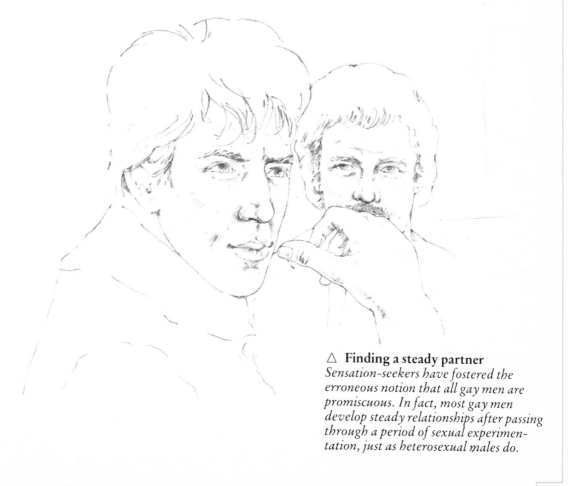

△ **Finding a steady partner**
Sensation-seekers have fostered the erroneous notion that all gay men are promiscuous. In fact, most gay men develop steady relationships after passing through a period of sexual experimentation, just as heterosexual males do.

ORIENTATION PROBLEMS

Most men have a strong sense of their own maleness, and find it easy to conform to the stereotype of masculinity. But this view of the male as the active, aggressive, dominant partner in any relationship is falling out of favor with both men and women. For both sexes there is great satisfaction in a merging of sexual roles so that however confident they are in their own masculinity, men are free to develop the 'feminine' qualities of caring and tenderness rather than cling to a restrictive 'macho' image.

Gender conflicts
A few men have problems because they lack an innate sense of being male. This makes it difficult for them to play a masculine role. There is a conflict between their 'core' gender – the sex they feel themselves to be – and their evident maleness. They may feel real only when they dress or behave as women.

Transvestism
The practice of dressing as a member of the opposite sex is known as transvestism. It is probably not rare but, because of the secrecy it involves, there can be no authoritative estimate of the number of men who practise it. Some men, known as fetishistic transvestites, cross-dress because they find wearing women's clothes sexually arousing. It may provide the special stimulation they need or it may be an end in itself, providing sexual satisfaction whether or not a partner is involved.

In many cases, though, the transvestite cross-dresses simply because he feels more at ease, more wholly himself, when dressed as a woman. It may be that he cross-dresses only in the privacy of his own home. Alternatively, he may try to pass as a woman in public, and, if so, much of his satisfaction will come from the success with which he does this. Often a transvestite can maintain a double life, with distinct male and female personalities, for years. But occasionally a transvestite's desire to play a female role becomes so intense that he decides he wants to *be* a woman rather than simply dress as one (see **Transsexualism**, opposite).

Homosexual transvestism
Most transvestites are heterosexual and about three quarters marry and have children. A small group of homosexuals, however, are effeminate in appearance and behavior and may cross-dress to reinforce these traits. But while the true transvestite will go to a great deal of trouble to look as much like a real woman as possible, the homosexual 'queen' will go over the top in his impersonation, creating a caricature rather than a realistic image of womanhood.

Coming to terms with transvestism
Very few male transvestites see their desire to cross-dress as an 'illness' or seek medical treatment unless there is marital or family pressure on them to do so. There is, in any case, no specific treatment to 'cure' the condition (though if you are determined that this is what you want, some kinds of behavior therapy may help, especially with fetishistic transvestism). But, as a general rule, if you consult a doctor you will be offered help with specific problems such as the effect on your marriage.

Marriage and transvestism
Many women can accept their partner's need to cross-dress, especially if it is occasional and discreet. But the more determined you are to develop and enhance your feminine side, the more strain you are likely to put on your relationship. If you value your partner, you will try to make cross-dressing a less important part of your life.

If you have not yet established what you hope will be a long-lasting relationship, but want to do so, you should think about the impact your cross-dressing is likely to have on your life with a partner. The following course of action is recommended once you have decided to confront the problem. Tell your partner about your cross-dressing before you are both fully committed to the relationship. If you do not tell her in advance she will feel even more cheated if she discovers at a later date and will then find it much harder to accept, having become used to you as a 'normal' male.

If your partner can accept what you have told her, try to agree on limits to your future cross-dressing, and you may in time be able to reduce the habit still further. Alternatively, your partner may feel able to cope provided she is not involved and you keep that part of your life separate. Or you may agree to cross-dress at home but never in public or in company. If you are very fortunate, your partner may be prepared to give you advice on clothes and make-up and let you play the feminine role at least some of the time.

Most countries have organizations (see RE-SOURCE GUIDE, p.156) which not only give support and counseling to transvestites, but provide opportunities for them to meet others and cross-dress in company without running the risks involved in doing so in public.

Transsexualism

For a very small number of men cross-dressing is not enough. This kind of man does not simply want to look and act like a woman, but to *be* one. The transsexual, as he is known, is convinced, despite possessing male genitals, that he is in fact a woman. Sometimes he will manage to lead a reasonably contented double life, but often he will seek surgery to become as nearly female as possible. Unlike transvestites, transsexuals seldom marry.

Treatment for the transsexual

The ultimate goal for the transsexual man is a sex-change operation. However, when he first consults a doctor, the latter will almost certainly suggest other solutions before allowing him to undergo irreversible surgery. He may recommend that his patient tries to carry on living the dual-life of the transvestite, for example. Or, if he has a male partner already, in anticipation of a sex change, the patient may be advised to test whether both he and his partner can accept and feel as comfortable with this kind of relationship as with a homosexual one.

Preparing for a sex change

If you feel strongly that a sex change is the only answer for you, you will be expected to spend at least 18 months living and supporting yourself as a woman before surgery is considered. You are likely to meet many problems that cannot be solved by surgery and this period will give you a chance to decide whether you will be able to cope with them. Meanwhile, practical steps, such as those listed below, will be suggested to help you develop your feminine side and make it easier for you to pass as a woman. It may be that you find these are enough and that you decide to put aside the idea of surgery.

☐ Avoid the temptation to be over-feminine in your dress and make-up. Padding and corseting, for example, may produce a figure that seems feminine to you, but will look like a caricature to others. You will do better to be more unobtrusive. Remember too that by day most women dress casually and wear little make-up. The sort of effect you may be striving for would probably look out of place except on a film set.

☐ Hormonal treatment may be given, but it will not work miracles. It will make your hips and thighs more feminine and rounded, your face fuller, and your skin softer. But it will not enlarge the breasts very much, or alter your voice or the male pattern of hair distribution on the face and body.

☐ Electrolysis removes facial hair permanently, but it takes many treatments over about five years.

☐ Training with a therapist will help you learn the social skills involved in being a woman.

Sex-change operations

In a male-to-female sex change, a vagina is modeled from the skin of the penis and scrotum. Complications are quite common, but if the operation is successful the subject is able to have intercourse as a woman, and may enjoy pleasurable sensations and even orgasm. However, sometimes so much reliance is placed on the results of surgery that its effects come as an anticlimax and lead to severe depression. A sex-change operation does not, of course, enable the recipient to have children, nor to be legally married as a woman.

BISEXUALITY

Gay men sometimes develop heterosexual relationships at the same time as having homosexual ones, and some marry. A substantial number of straight men have homosexual experiences in adolescence, particularly if living in an all-male environment, and a few have similar encounters when their marriage is under stress or their partner is pregnant. Some men are more truly bisexual; they can enjoy sexual relationships with both men and women, though they are not always equally responsive to either sex. The true bisexual may try to present his more socially acceptable heterosexual side. He may also have to contend with the homosexual's view that bisexuality is a refusal to choose.

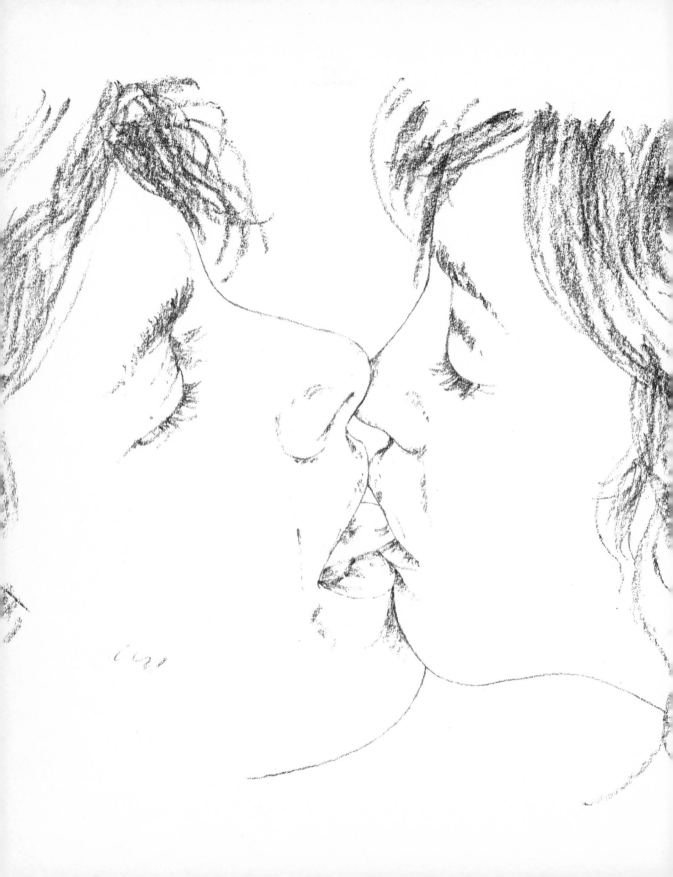

4

THE MAN WITH A STEADY PARTNER

Being part of a couple implies emotional commitment as well as sexual attachment and most couples prefer their relationship to be sexually exclusive. Monogamy is still the ideal most people strive for, even if it is not always achieved, and they expect of it both emotional security and physical satisfaction. Many of the problems you will face as a couple and which are discussed in this part of the book will arise simply because you have made this commitment to each other. They seem to be the most inescapable facts of a shared life. Few long-term partners will not experience, at some time or other, the overfamiliarity that can lead to boredom, or at least to a sexual wistfulness. Many will experience jealousy, or have to deal with the threat of infidelity.

The final section of this part of the book deals with contraception, with the problems of the couple who want to have a child but have so far been unable to, and offers guidance to the man whose partner is pregnant or has recently given birth.

COMPATIBILITY

Being compatible as a couple means being able to live together in a pleasurable and satisfying way. This is possible when your personalities and viewpoints are reasonably similar or complement each other so well that there is seldom serious conflict between you. The qualities that make for compatibility in a relationship are discussed more fully in MAKING A LASTING RELATIONSHIP, p.144.

Yet it is quite possible to live together happily even though you may not seem, in theory, altogether compatible. Indeed no couple who live together for any length of time will see eye to eye on every issue, or always have the same needs at the same time. As important and valuable as compatibility of temperament is being able to deal with issues as they arise and to resolve them by making the necessary shifts of attitude before the whole relationship is jeopardized.

If you can do this, it will benefit your sex life as well as your overall happiness. The couple who get along well in other ways and who are loving and committed to each other will not normally allow sexual differences or difficulties to sour their whole relationship. Sex therapists have found, too, that while most sexual problems can be resolved successfully if a couple's general relationship is close and loving, therapy is less likely to succeed if there is hostility between the people involved.

Certain areas of a shared life are especially vital to the wellbeing of a relationship, while others are abundant sources of discontent. The questionnaire that follows explores these crucial areas, allowing you to see how well you have adjusted to each other's needs. You can answer on your own, but it is better to both do it, each keeping your own score.

HOW WELL DO YOU SUIT EACH OTHER?

1 How much of your leisure time do you spend with your partner?

Most	2
Some	1
Little or none	0

2 How many of your friends are mutual friends whose company you both enjoy?

Few or none	0
Most	2
Some	1

3 If your partner wants to spend a quiet evening at home together do you usually:

Welcome and enjoy it?	2
Not mind?	1
Feel bored?	0

4 If you have dinner in a restaurant with just your partner do you find:

It is a good opportunity to talk?	2
You have got very little to say to each other?	0
It is quite pleasant but not stimulating?	1

5 If your work (or your partner's) began to limit your time together would you:

Try to alter your timetable?	2
Decide there was little you could do?	1
Welcome it?	0

6 Of your three main interests how many does your partner share?

One or two	1
All three	2
None	0

7 How often do you vacation together?

Always	2
Usually	1
Rarely	0

8 If your partner is clearly worried about something, does she usually:

Refuse to talk about it?	0
Discuss it with you?	2
Talk about it if you press her?	1

9 When you talk about what you have been doing, thinking, or feeling, how often does your partner seem interested?

Sometimes _____ 1
Always _____ 2
Seldom _____ 0

10 Do disagreements with your partner most often lead to:

Discussion? _____ 2
A spirited argument? _____ 1
Serious or prolonged hostility? _____ 0

11 How often do you quarrel fiercely over trivial issues?

Often _____ 0
Seldom or never _____ 2
Occasionally _____ 1

12 Are you ever concerned because your partner is much more of a spendthrift (or more careful with money) than you are?

Never _____ 2
Sometimes _____ 1
Continually _____ 0

13 If an expensive item is needed for use by both of you (a car or furniture, for example) how often do you have what you consider a fair say in choosing it?

Sometimes _____ 1
Always _____ 2
Seldom or never _____ 0

14 Do you feel you have less say than you would like in deciding how unallocated money is spent?

No, I am happy with the situation _____ 2
Yes, I would like more say _____ 1
What I would like is seldom considered _____ 0

15 Do you agree with your partner on domestic expenditure?

Not at all _____ 0
Completely _____ 2
The situation could be better _____ 1

16 Do you ever feel lonely or resentful because your partner seems to have a greater need for solitude than you do?

Seldom or never _____ 2
Sometimes _____ 1
Often _____ 0

17 Does your partner 'crowd' you so that you have little or no time for yourself?

Most of the time _____ 0
Seldom or never _____ 2
Sometimes _____ 1

18 Would you like to spend more time doing things without your partner?

Not at all _____ 2
A little more _____ 1
Much more _____ 0

19 How often do problems arise because your partner resents you seeing other people or doing things without her?

Occasionally _____ 1
Seldom or never _____ 2
Often _____ 0

20 How often does jealousy cause problems between you?

Seldom or never _____ 2
Occasionally _____ 1
Often _____ 0

21 Do you feel that your partner's parents loom too large in your life, that you spend too much time with them, or that her views about things that only concern the two of you are too much influenced by theirs?

Not at all _____ 2
A little _____ 1
Very much _____ 0

22 Do you wish that your partner's approach to work was:

More ambitious? _____ 0
Less ambitious? _____ 0
Neither _____ 2

23 Does your job ever disrupt your time together?

Seldom	2
Often	0
Sometimes	1

24 Does your partner's job ever disrupt your time together?

Sometimes	1
Often	0
Seldom	2

25 Do you and your partner agree about a woman's right to work if she wants to?

Completely	2
With reservations	1
Not at all	0

26 If you have no children, do you and your partner agree about whether or when to start a family?

With reservations	1
Not at all	0
Completely	2

27 If you have children, do you feel that your partner's attitude toward their rearing is:

About right?	2
Too strict?	0
Too easygoing?	0

28 Have you ever seriously considered ending your relationship?

Often	0
Never	2
Once or twice	1

RATING

High rating (36-56)

This suggests that you are content in your relationship, and that it meets most, if not all, of your emotional needs. You probably feel you have room to grow within it too, even though it gives you the support and security you currently need.

Medium rating (25-35)

This indicates that you probably get on well enough for your relationship to have a good chance of permanence. However, if you scored low in a particular group of questions, consult the detailed analysis of the questions, below.

Low rating (0-24)

This suggests that dissatisfaction with your day-to-day life is likely to spill over into your sex life. Couples who argue a lot tend to have a less active and less satisfying sex life. Look through your answers to discover where the major difficulties lie. Does your partner score low on the same questions? If so, you probably both need to make adjustments in those areas. If there is a discrepancy between your scores, it may be that one partner is making *all* the adjustments. In this case the low-scoring partner may need to be a little more assertive if you are to achieve a more balanced and satisfying relationship.

ANALYSIS OF THE QUESTIONS

Questions 1-7 deal with companionship.
Companionship is one of the most important things you can give each other. A 1983 survey of American couples indicated that couples who spend little of their time together are less satisfied and therefore more liable to break up than more companionable couples.

You are more likely to be happy and to develop a more intimate relationship if you have mutual friends and interests. If you spend too much time away from each other you risk loosening the bonds of intimacy. The main danger for the couple who spend little of their free time together is that they may come to find that most of the time they do spend together is concerned largely with resolving domestic problems, particularly those involving money. Since these are certainly the least appealing aspects of a shared life, their relationship will grow less and less rewarding and there may seem to be little reason to make strenuous efforts to sustain it.

Companionship seems to be an area in which the homosexual couple often scores over the heterosexual. Gay couples are more likely to have interests and leisure activities in common than are heterosexual couples. It is usually worthwhile for the heterosexual couple to seek activities that interest them both and to make an attempt to enjoy more leisure time together.

Questions 8-11 deal with communication.

For many couples, problems arise simply because they do not talk to each other enough, or because they talk without actually communicating much, keeping each other at an emotional distance so that real feelings are seldom shared and misunderstandings inevitably occur. Some people expect from their partner an almost telepathic ability to communicate, because the words they use bear little relation to the message they really want to convey. For example, complaints are directed at easy targets ('You never put the cat out when it's your turn') when the real source of dissatisfaction ('You're not as loving as I'd like you to be') is harder both to recognize and to put into words. If you often have quarrels about trivial things that grow out of all proportion, it usually indicates a much deeper dissatisfaction – about lack of love, or security, or companionship – which you must both confront.

For some couples, feelings of anger cause the most problems. Many people are afraid of showing anger because they feel it will inevitably bring the whole relationship down around their ears. There is at least some foundation for this fear since if you often get very angry it can be enormously destructive of your relationship. Marriage guidance counselors find that anger frequently heads the list of one partner's complaints about the other. However, things are little better if you do not show anger at all, because the problems that caused it may then never be acknowledged or resolved. The tension and resentment that build up within you can be equally destructive. The advice in **Dealing with anger**, p.115, will help you contain and defuse an angry situation before it can do too much damage.

Questions 12-15 concern money.

Most studies report that between one quarter and one third of all couples quarrel more about money than about anything else. It is not only lack of money that affects a couple's contentment (though it is important, and the less there is, the more fights there are likely to be about it) but also the questions of who should earn it and how it should be spent. Arguments about money are also arguments about trust, about

commitment to the relationship, about interdependence or equality. So if money is what you tend to fight about, discover which of these issues are really at stake and deal with them.

Married couples usually pool their resources, often sharing a bank account, to show their trust in and commitment to each other. Couples who live together often try, at least to begin with, to maintain separate finances, which certainly gives them one less issue to quarrel about. By doing this they are also, perhaps unconsciously, ensuring that the ties between them will be easier to dissolve if necessary.

Sharing money shows faith in a future together, and indeed almost every couple, heterosexual or homosexual, who have been together for any length of time do this as their commitment grows and the financial strings of their lives become more entwined. But problems can arise if they have different attitudes toward money. If one partner is easy-come, easy-go, while the other is a prudent saver for a rainy day, for example, there may be difficulties; likewise if the partner who is the higher (or the only) earner feels he or she should exercise far greater or even total control over expenditure.

Questions 16-21 are about privacy and independence.

However close you are, you will probably feel the need for some privacy from your partner. This is a need that seems to be more pressing for women than for men. Couples who live together usually regard private time and personal space as more important than couples who marry, because they feel that independence within the relationship is essential. Every couple has to find the balance between independence and separateness that suits them best. Problems can occur if either partner has an excessive need for privacy or independence because this is likely to affect the time they spend together, which is one of the most important elements binding them. Even so, too much togetherness can be smothering. Life may be equally unsatisfactory for a couple if one partner is so dependent on the other for emotional support and company that he or she allows the other no breathing space.

Arguments about in-laws are often arguments about dependence, about whether a partner has really achieved the necessary emotional break with his or her parents and made a total commitment to the relationship. Such a partner may insist on living close to his or her parents, visiting them unreasonably often, taking their side in an argument against the other partner, and consulting them automatically on every important decision that affects the couple.

Questions 22-25 examine how your work affects the relationship.
Dissatisfaction here is often about the inroads one partner's job makes on the time you might otherwise spend together. But probably the most serious arguments arise in couples who have not agreed about a woman's right to work or about the extent of her commitment to her work. This problem is among those most likely to break up a relationship.

Ambition affects significantly the way you feel about each other. While women like their partners to be ambitious and successful, men – unless they are very confident and successful themselves – are usually less happy about having an ambitious partner.

Questions 26 and 27 concern your attitudes toward parenthood.
Most studies suggest that children are by no means indispensable to a couple's happiness, even that life together is more fulfilling for the childless couple. Where there are children, the most frequent disagreements in the sphere of parenthood concern, as might be expected, the basics of their rearing and the particularly difficult question of discipline. However, if you can genuinely develop, or at least present to the children, a united front on these issues, you will avoid a major source of potential conflict.

Question 28 concerns the fundamental stability of your relationship.
Nearly everybody feels like walking out on his or her partner at times. But if you have frequently taken this course of action, only to return, or even if you merely contemplate if often, then the relationship is clearly not working. Your reasons for planning a separation are almost certainly pinpointed by your answers to the rest of this questionnaire. Study the detailed analysis of the other questions.

Lasting compatibility ▷
The willingness to confront problems in a relationship and to be flexible about their resolution is indispensable to long-term compatibility.

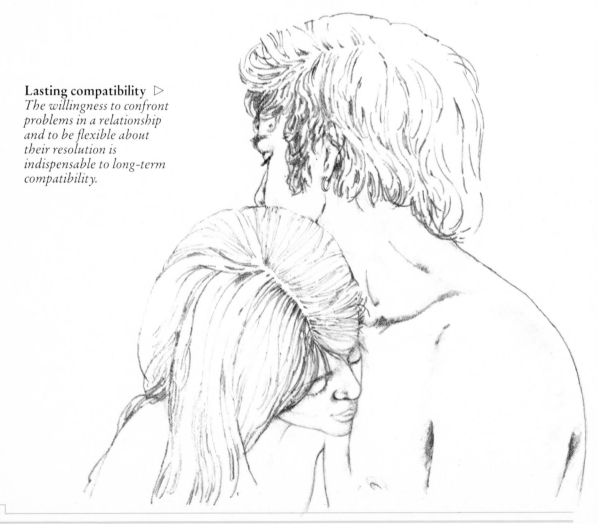

ARE YOU SEXUALLY SATISFIED?

Sex is one of the strongest ties that can hold two people together, and it is a bond that you can foster and strengthen by making sure that your sex life is as satisfying as possible for both of you. The questionnaire below deals with some of the most important elements of sexual satisfaction, and it should provide a measure of your contentment with this aspect of your relationship. You can do the questionnaire alone, or better still, with your partner, keeping separate scores. The results will indicate your sexual compatibility and show whether there is a particularly problematic area.

DO YOU SATISFY EACH OTHER SEXUALLY?

1 Do you have sex:

As often as you want? _____ 2
Not often enough? _____ 0
Too often for your taste? _____ 0

2 Do you find your partner attractive?

Very _____ 2
Fairly _____ 1
Not very _____ 0

3 Who usually initiates sex?

The male partner _____ 1
The female partner _____ 0
Either partner _____ 2

4 Is the 'refusal rate' (when one partner suggests sex):

More or less equal? _____ 2
Very unequal? _____ 0

5 If your partner says no to sex, do you:

Feel rejected, hurt, or angry, and keep a mental note of it? _____ 0
Feel briefly irritated or disappointed? _____ 1
Accept that she or he is not in the mood? _____ 2

6 If you say no to sex, does your partner:

Get angry or upset? _____ 0
Seem briefly disappointed or annoyed? _____ 1
Understand that you are just not in the mood? _____ 2

7 Do you wish your partner was:

Less prudish or inhibited about sex? _____ 0
Less fond of sexual experimentation? _____ 0
Neither _____ 2

8 Do you get enough affection during sex?

Always _____ 2
Mostly _____ 1
Never _____ 0

9 Do you get affection outside of sex?

Always _____ 2
Never _____ 0
Mostly _____ 1

10 How often does your partner want you to try a sexual activity you dislike?

Seldom or never _____ 2
Sometimes _____ 1
Often _____ 0

11 Do you have erection problems (or does your partner have vaginal problems) that make sex difficult or impossible?

Seldom or never _____ 2
Sometimes _____ 1
Often _____ 0

12 Is sex unsatisfactory because you (or your partner) fail to reach orgasm:

Sometimes? _____ 1
Never? _____ 0
Seldom or never? _____ 2

13 How often is sex unsatisfactory for you because you (or your partner) reach orgasm too quickly?

Seldom or never _____ 2
Sometimes _____ 1
Often _____ 0

14 How often is sex unsatisfactory for you because your partner just does not seem interested?

Seldom or never _____ 2
Sometimes _____ 1
Often _____ 0

15 Has either of you had sex outside the relationship?

Within the last year _____ 0
Since the relationship began _____ 1
Never _____ 2

16 Is sex with your partner as varied as you would like it to be?

Yes _____ 2
Not quite as varied _____ 1
Not at all _____ 0

17 How often do you (or does your partner) pick quarrels at bedtime?

Often _____ 0
Occasionally _____ 1
Seldom or never _____ 2

18 How often do you go to bed long before or long after your partner?

Always _____ 0
Sometimes _____ 1
Seldom or never _____ 2

19 Do you suggest sex when it is hard for your partner to respond because of a task that cannot be left?

Often _____ 0
Sometimes _____ 1
Seldom or never _____ 2

20 How often, if sex seems imminent, do you begin to recall past grievances so that you feel resentment toward your partner?

Often _____ 0
Seldom or never _____ 2
Sometimes _____ 1

RATING

High rating (26-40)
This shows that your present relationship meets your sexual needs very well. You most likely get along well with your partner in other ways, because sexual satisfaction is a good indicator of the quality of your relationship.

Medium rating (16-25)
This indicates that you have worked out a sexual relationship that suits both partners. However, you will probably both acknowledge that there is scope for improvement. Consult the detailed analysis below about questions for which your score was low.

Low rating (0-15)
This suggests a lack of satisfaction with either the quality or the quantity of your sex life, or both. However, checking through the detailed analysis below will help you to establish, and then set about dispelling, the principal causes of dissatisfaction. If you scored low on questions 17-20, and especially if your score on the preceding questionnaire was also low, your lack of sexual contentment may reflect a disharmony in other areas of your relationship. Clearing up difficulties which may be marring your everyday life together will almost certainly lead to greater enjoyment of sex for both of you.

ANALYSIS OF THE QUESTIONS

*Question **1** deals with sexual frequency.*

For most couples, good sex means frequent sex. Couples who have sex infrequently report less overall satisfaction than couples who make love often. It is easy for your sex life to become pared down without either of you fully realizing it. You may, for example, get into a routine of not having sex at a time when one or other of you is tired or busy, and then find that it is not easy to break the habit and establish a new pattern of wanting sex and making time for it. If either of you fails to score on this question, it may be because there is a sex-drive discrepancy between you (see DEALING WITH A SEX-DRIVE DISCREPANCY, p.116). But it may simply be because you have stopped giving sex the priority in your lives that it deserves.

*Question **2** concerns sexual attraction.*

For this there is no real explanation and certainly no substitute. Finding your partner attractive seems to be one of the most important factors in determining how satisfying your sex life is. You cannot create this sexual chemistry if it does not exist, but you can foster and sustain it when it is present by not taking each other for granted or abandoning all efforts to be attractive to your partner.

*Questions **3-6** deal with the sharing of sexual responsibility.*

Traditionally, the man suggests sex and the woman either accepts or rejects him, so usually it is the former who determines how much sex the couple have. Couples seem to be happiest, and to have sex most often, when both partners feel equally free to suggest sex or to refuse it, and do so equally often. If you can share control of sex like this you are much less likely to feel angry or rejected if you want sex and your partner does not, or to feel guilty on the occasions when she feels like it and you do not. Inclination rather than obligation will then determine how often you have sex.

*Questions **7-10**, **14** and **16** concern your sexual compatibility.*

As in most other areas of your life together, the more similar your sexual likes and dislikes are, the less friction there will be between you. If either of you scores low in this section, you will find EXPANDING YOUR SEXUAL REPERTOIRE, p.48 and UNDERSTANDING A WOMAN'S FEELINGS, p.117, helpful.

*Questions **11-13** deal with specific sexual problems.*

Such problems will inevitably affect the quality of your sexual relationship. If the problem is your own, the relevant features will help. If it is your partner who has a sexual problem, reading **The female orgasm**, p.118, together will probably be helpful to both of you.

*Question **15** concerns infidelity.*

This is much more likely to be a symptom of dissatisfaction with your relationship than a cause of it. INFIDELITY, p.124, suggests ways of minimizing the damage to your relationship that this situation will almost certainly cause.

*Questions **17-20** deal with sexual sabotage.*

If your score in this section is low, sex may be unsatisfying because it has become a weapon you use against each other instead of a source of mutual pleasure. You may be using it as a punishment, withholding it to perpetuate a quarrel or to get even for past grievances. Or you may be using it to make your partner feel inadequate or guilty by always suggesting you make love when it is obviously impossible or inconvenient. If you find that you have reduced your sex life to a minimum by this kind of sabotage, there is sure to be more wrong with your relationship than just sex. Your answers to the preceding questionnaire, on compatibility, may help you discover the underlying problem.

WHAT IS WRONG WITH YOUR RELATIONSHIP?

Is it sex that causes the biggest problems between you?

YES →

Is the main problem a difference of sex drive, so that you want sex much more (or less) often than your partner?

YES →

See DEALING WITH A SEX-DRIVE DISCREPANCY, p.116.

NO ↓

Does your partner seem uninterested in sex, making it hard for you to arouse her?

YES →

See **Women and sexual satisfaction**, p.117.

NO ↓

See **The female orgasm**, p.118.

Are you concerned because your partner does not easily or often reach orgasm?

YES →

NO ↓

Is your sex life temporarily unsatisfactory because sex is painful for your partner?

YES →

See **Painful intercourse**, p.120.

NO ↓

Does your partner seem to have a strong dislike or fear of sex?

YES →

Does she feel that she is 'too small', so that her vagina tightens and intercourse becomes difficult or impossible?

NO ↓

NO ←   **YES** ↓

Your partner's inhibitions about sex may stem from an upbringing which made her feel it was 'dirty' or wrong. If you can encourage her to talk about her feelings, you will probably be better able to understand how she feels and perhaps even help her develop a more positive attitude toward sex.

See **Fear of penetration**, p.119.

NO ↓

NO **NO**

Is your problem one of differing sexual tastes, so that you like to do some things your partner regards as perverted (or vice versa)?

YES → See **Conflicting sexual tastes**, p.120.

NO

Do you feel that you have been with your partner for so long that sex has become predictable and boring?

YES → See AVOIDING SEXUAL BOREDOM, p.122.

NO

Answer the questionnaire ARE YOU SEXUALLY SATISFIED?, p.109. This may disclose other areas of incompatibility or specific problems that are making your relationship unsatisfactory.

Does jealousy often cause problems between you?

YES → Is there a real basis for this? Have you or (to your knowledge) your partner been unfaithful?

YES → See INFIDELITY, p.124.

NO

NO

See JEALOUSY, p.126.

DANGER SIGNS

Below are the most common symptoms of a relationship that is running into serious trouble. If any of them applies to yours, answer the questionnaires COMPATIBILITY, p.104, and ARE YOU SEXUALLY SATISFIED?, p.109, to find possible causes of the tension between you.

☐ Frequent arguments over trivial matters

☐ Apathy and boredom

☐ Loss of sexual interest

☐ Failure of one or both partners to listen to and understand the other's complaints

See the questionnaire COMPATIBILITY, p.104, which explores some of the most common reasons for a couple's difficulty in living pleasurably together.

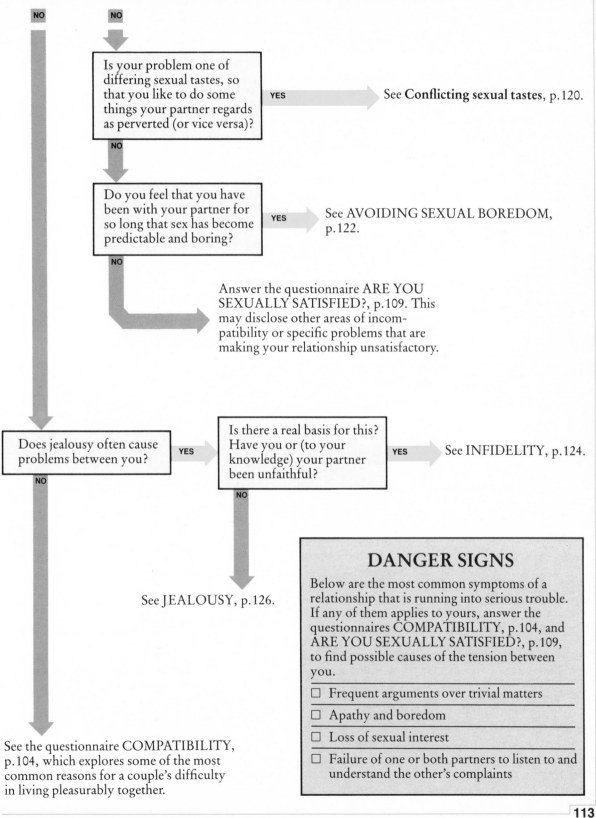

LEARNING TO COMMUNICATE

Talking about sex in a general way interests nearly everybody, but few find it easy to discuss personal reactions and sexual preferences. Sharing intimate thoughts and feelings with a partner means revealing private areas of oneself, and this makes many men needlessly uncomfortable.

Talking about sex

Gestures – a hug in the right place at the right time, for example – can say a lot, but without words they can be misunderstood. Do not expect your partner to be able to read your mind, for it is a fallacy to believe that if she cares for you she will know what you want. There is no substitute for straight talking if you want to discover what you both need.

Take advantage of a new relationship by starting to discuss your preferences, and encouraging your partner to discuss hers, as soon as you begin to have sex. It is often much easier to talk intimately to someone you do not know well than to break an established routine and start talking to a long-term lover with whom you have always found it difficult to talk about sex.

Communicate directly, and be as specific as you can. Do not just say, 'How was that?' Say, 'Did I get the pressure right?' or 'Was I touching you in the right place?' or 'Was it too fast for you?' And say straight out what *you* would like to do or not do, what *you* want or do not want. If you try to guess your partner's likes and dislikes and behave as you believe she prefers, you may guess wrong. And if both of you play this game, neither of you is likely to get what you want. So be direct and encourage your partner to be the same.

Reassuring your partner

Give reassurance and encouragement whenever you can. It probably works better (at least until you are quite confident of the relationship) to stress what you like rather than complain about what you dislike. So say, 'That feels great,' rather than 'I don't much like what you're doing now'. Comments beginning 'You never ....' or 'You always ....' convey criticism of a partner's ability in bed and usually make for tension.

You should be particularly tactful if you want to introduce a topic that is clearly sensitive, such as personal hygiene. One approach is to suggest that the problem may be one you share. Ask her to check your breath, for example, and to tell you if it is bad. It is then reasonable for you to do the same. Or tell her you have not taken a bath for a couple of days and suggest you shower together before bed.

Giving or demanding complete self-exposure all at once can make your partner back off if she is not ready for it. Never ask a question you would not be willing to answer yourself or one that you are sure will deeply embarrass your partner.

The right time to talk

For most men the best time to start talking about sex is during lovemaking. Try to be appreciative, letting your partner know what you like while you are enjoying it. Try also to be discreetly inquisitive. Ask your partner, 'Do you like that?' or 'Shall I go on with it?' Let her feel that you will respond to whatever hints she might like to make. At the same time, casually mention your own preferences.

Some men, though, find it easier to bring up the subject of sexual preferences at other times. This is likely to be the case if you are involved in a long-standing relationship in which you and your partner have not been in the habit of talking about sex. Try introducing the subject when you are on neutral ground – over a drink or a meal, for example, when you should both feel comfortable and relaxed. And broach it indirectly, by means of something you have read or seen on TV, or even by quoting a friend's experience.

Reliving pleasurable experiences

It is usually easier, too, to talk in terms of past experience rather than about the present. If you wish you could repeat a certain kind of sexual activity that you once enjoyed together, speak of it reminiscently as a pleasurable experience, as this can lead to a suggestion that you do it again. It may help if you rehearse what you are going to say in advance. Working out the wording and saying it aloud to yourself will increase your confidence when you broach the subject with your partner.

Saying no

For many men, one of the most difficult communication problems is finding a way of telling a partner that you are just not in the mood for sex without making her feel rejected. You yourself undoubtedly know how hurt and rejected you can feel because of a sexual rebuff. It is important to learn how to reject the invitation without rejecting the person. You could, for example, say, 'I'd love to sit and talk for a while but I'm just not in the mood for sex tonight'. Or you might decline gently and say, 'Why don't we just have a cuddle?'

Many couples who find it difficult to be forthright prefer to adopt a code to convey sexual readiness. You might agree on a 0-10 scale, for example. Then, if either of you says, 'Sorry, but I rate zero tonight', the other knows this means total unwillingness. On the other hand, a 3 or 4 might mean 'I can probably make it if you're really keen.' Or you could choose a code based on appetite, ranging from 'I could eat a horse' down to 'All I need is a cup of black coffee'.

A code system prevents the development of 'heavy' situations fraught with misunderstanding. It makes it clear that you are just talking about a temporary mood. The number code, in particular, allows for maneuver. If one of you is an 8, for example, while the other shows a flicker of interest with a 3, the person with the lower rating might be prepared to make an extra effort for the sake of the more highly aroused partner. As long as you agree on the respective values of the code words, the second system might also be used in this way.

Learn to listen

It is easy to forget that listening properly is as important as communicating your own feelings. Show that you are listening by looking at your partner when she is talking. You can still listen buried in the newspaper, but it does not look like it. Make appropriate listening noises also: 'Uh huh, tell me more, how did you feel about that . . . ' It is a good idea, too, to paraphrase what she has said before responding: 'They seem to have given you a hard time at work today then. No wonder you are feeling so low . . . ', to show that you have really understood what is being said.

Picking up non-verbal cues

Pay particular attention to what your partner does to you during sexual encounters. You can usually assume that when she emphasizes a gesture she wants to enjoy the same thing. Such non-verbal cues are the easiest way for some people to let their partners know their sexual preferences. So if she should suck your nipples or fondle your genitals or anus, the chances are strong that reciprocation would be very welcome.

Dealing with anger

For nearly everyone anger and good sex are incompatible. In any relationship, especially a long-term one, quarrels and hurt feelings should be dealt with as they arise, not left to fester. Suppressed resentment contributes to sexual problems and makes them increasingly hard to resolve.

It is important for any couple, particularly those with sexual problems that they are trying to surmount, to be able to deal with anger. Occasional episodes of unpleasantness are bound to arise in nearly every relationship, but they can be resolved without lasting bitterness if the partners can talk over without delay the real cause of the trouble. Here are some guidelines for a sensible approach to such situations:

☐ Tell your partner exactly what has upset you, and do it at the time, not a week later.

☐ Deal with the problem in terms of your own feelings rather than your partner's behavior. Say, 'Perhaps I shouldn't get angry when . . . but I do' rather than 'You're so selfish, you don't ever . . .'.

☐ Stick to the particular issue and resolve it. Do not use the present argument as an opportunity to get past resentments off your chest.

☐ Exercise self-control, no matter how irritated you are. Arguments should not be damaging or destructive. So, if you are so angry that you feel like shouting at or hitting your partner, wait until the white heat of your rage dies down before tackling the issue.

☐ Do not make wounding attacks on each other's physical or intellectual shortcomings as these are not easily forgotten or forgiven.

☐ The moment an argument seems to be degenerating into a destructive fight, give it up and suggest that you would rather resolve it later when you both feel calmer.

☐ Make it up before bedtime, or as soon as you get into bed, but never try to use sex to make up after a fight. Most women are very turned off by this and the rift then takes even longer to heal.

DEALING WITH A SEX-DRIVE DISCREPANCY

Couples often wonder about how often they should be having sex, as though they are somehow failing if they fall behind the probable average of about 2.5 times a week. But quoting averages is pointless, since all that matters is that you should make love as much, or as little, as you both want.

It is part of the widespread 'macho' ideal that a man should always be interested in and ready for sex. Consequently, if sex has never been important to you, or if you suddenly find you have less drive than usual, you may start to harbor doubts about your masculinity.

A few men even believe the old myth, perpetuated by sports coaches who feel that sexual abstinence will magically put an edge on a sportsman's performance, that 'too much' sex weakens a man. It does not. Never be influenced by the notion that sex is a competitive sport.

Fluctuating sexual appetite

Like any other appetite, your sexual needs will wax and wane, and various factors make it perfectly natural to lack desire. The most crucial of these is your feeling toward your partner. If you are no longer attracted to her, or have a relationship that is fraught with anger or resentment, then your sex drive is likely to be low, or even non-existent.

Again, if you are depressed, for example, you will probably have little interest in sex. And it is natural for your sex drive to decrease when you are physically ill and to subside a little in later life too.

Inhibitions and your sex drive

If you have always had a low sex drive, it is possible that the way you were raised, or a traumatic experience with sex when you were young, has so inhibited you that you have always suppressed that part of your feelings, perhaps even avoiding sex altogether. If this is the case you should find OVERCOMING INHIBITIONS, p.68, helpful.

A high or low sex drive becomes a problem only when it differs very greatly from your partner's. This is a difficulty which is likely to be more serious if your own drive is much lower than your partner's, partly because of the general assumption that men should initiate sex, and partly because it is easier, physically, for a woman to have intercourse when not aroused than it is for a man.

Bridging a sex-drive gap

However, a sex-drive discrepancy need not mean that one of you is continually frustrated. Listed below are some of the most effective ways in which you can sustain a close and loving sexual relationship when intercourse is not as frequent as the more highly sexed partner would wish.

☐ Remember that sex need not involve intercourse. Even if you are not aroused yourself, you can use manual and oral stimulation to satisfy your partner (see STIMULATION TECHNIQUES, p.50) or give each other the relaxing pleasure of skillful caresses (see LEARNING TO SHARE PLEASURE, p.79).

☐ Many men feel that desire should be spontaneous, that they should not need direct stimulation in order to become aroused. This is not the case and is even less so as you grow older. So let your partner arouse you.

☐ Use psychic stimulation: erotic books and magazines, or erotic films and videos, or fantasy.

☐ If masturbation by one partner, while being held by the other, suits you both it can prove a good way of achieving both satisfaction and closeness when the 'low-drive' partner does not want intercourse. However, it will not provide a solution on every occasion.

☐ If you are the 'low-drive' partner, when you masturbate alone try to do it to a fantasy image of your partner so that you come to associate her with your feelings of sexual arousal. Start by using your own favorite fantasy, whatever it is, gradually 'shaping' it to include an image of your partner as you become more aroused, so that she eventually becomes the main stimulus.

☐ Do not withhold affection from your partner, especially if your own lack of sexual interest has become an issue between you. You may be tempted to avoid bodily contact for fear that she will interpret a demonstration of affection as a sexual initiative, but if you do she will feel emotionally as well as physically rejected.

UNDERSTANDING A WOMAN'S FEELINGS

Among the most important contributions a man can make to his relationship with a woman are to understand how she feels about and responds to sex, and to look at sexual problems from her point of view. Because sex is such an intimate area of our lives we tend to take our partner's problems very personally. For example, if you have a temporary erection problem because you are tired or preoccupied, your partner, unless she understands you very well, may need reassurance that your body's lack of reaction is not her fault nor indeed anything to do with your feelings for her. The reverse is also true: you will be able to sympathize and perhaps help her with any problem she has if you can understand that it does not arise from her feelings about you. (Occasionally a problem will arise from her feelings about you, and it is important that you understand when this is the case.)

Women and sexual satisfaction

Lack of empathy between the sexes is often the result of the very different attitudes toward sex of men and women. For most men sex has to achieve the goals of erection and orgasm if it is to be fully satisfying, while women often value the feelings of closeness and tenderness as much as sexual excitement. Therefore, it is very easy (and very common) for a man to achieve his sexual goals without meeting his partner's real needs at all. This difference of outlook has great bearing on other aspects of your relationship and is explored more fully in **What makes a good lover?**, p.48. It explains why, for example, monogamy matters so much more to women than to men. To a woman, a sexual encounter may well represent a potential emotional involvement and therefore a threat to her principal relationship. When she has 'outside' sex, she is more likely to be looking for a special relationship than simply seeking variety. You may have difficulty convincing your partner that a casual sexual affair was just that and no more, because, for her, emotional commitment is such an important component of sex.

What is frigidity?

The term 'frigidity' has come to be used pejoratively, to imply not only that a 'frigid' woman does not like sex, but often that she does not like men. It is an easy defense for a man who has failed to interest or arouse a woman to decide that she is 'frigid' and so neatly transfer the blame to her.

Quite apart from being an unfair description, the term 'frigid' is an imprecise one, making no distinction between the different sexual problems that women can face. A woman may have a temporary lack of interest in sex, so that she does not easily become aroused, for example. She may enjoy sex but seldom reach orgasm, or she may have such an intense fear of penetration that intercourse is impossible. Very rarely does the problem stem from a total aversion to sex – the emotional coldness that is implicit in the word 'frigid'. But often, if a woman does have this type of problem, it may be exacerbated, or will at least remain unresolved, because her partner knows little about how a woman's sexuality differs from his own.

A woman's need of arousal

The major difference between a woman who is not sexually aroused and a man with an erection problem is that a woman can allow a man to make love to her without being excited herself, while a man cannot perform without the excitement that produces an erection. But having sex when she is not properly aroused will not be pleasurable for her and it may even be painful, because her vagina will fail to become adequately lubricated. And, if intercourse is forced upon her, she will almost certainly feel used.

Often, even if your partner does not seem to be interested in sex at first, you will be able to arouse her, but there may be times when she is particularly uninterested. A woman's sexual responsiveness (like a man's) varies from time to time. Many women find that their sexual desire is at its peak during menstruation, for example. Intercourse at this time is, despite a widespread belief to the contrary, harmless. Your partner may like to wear a diaphragm (if she uses one) when the flow is heavy, and a towel on the bed will take care of any leakage. Many of the things which affect your own level of interest or ability to get an erection will affect your partner too. These include physical and emotional illness, alcohol, and drugs (see problem charts LACK OF INTEREST, p.24, and ERECTION PROBLEMS, p.36). Listed on the following page are further factors that influence a woman's sexual arousal which both you and your partner should be aware of.

- Inadequate stimulation is the most obvious reason for a woman's failure to become aroused. If you are in too great a hurry for intercourse you may not be giving your partner the stimulation of her body, breasts, and genitals that she needs to arouse her. When she is excited her nipples will become erect, the vaginal lips and 'hood' of her clitoris will swell, her vagina will become wet and, when she is fully aroused, its lower part will swell and widen.

- The fear of pregnancy can lessen a woman's desire for sex. You can allay this fear by ensuring that you use a contraceptive technique that you both feel confident about (see CONTRACEPTION, p.127).

- Negative feelings about a partner have a profound effect on a woman's sexual response. Most women need to feel emotionally close to a partner to become aroused, and anger, hurt, or an unresolved quarrel normally make a woman far less responsive.

- Exhaustion frequently leads to a loss of sexual interest. The woman who faces the demands of the home, children, and perhaps a job as well, may simply not have the time and energy needed for good sex.

- Pain during intercourse inevitably makes it difficult for a woman to anticipate sex with pleasure (see **Painful intercourse**, p.120).

- Do not overlook the possibility that your partner's lack of interest, especially if it is longstanding, may be a reflection of a problem you yourself have. If sex has never been truly satisfying for her, perhaps because you reach orgasm too soon and then fall asleep, her disappointment may have gradually turned into a lack of interest.

The female orgasm

Both men and women are sometimes confused about the female orgasm. Your partner may worry about whether she has orgasms at all, and whether what she experiences is what she is supposed to feel. If she is not sure, you may feel it is your responsibility, while she may feel it is her failure. What ought to be simply a source of pleasure easily, and often unnecessarily, becomes a cause for concern. The following facts about the female orgasm may help both you and your partner if you have problems or gaps in your understanding in this area.

- The female orgasm is a series of intense pulsations within the vagina. Few women can reach orgasm through penetration alone. Unless a woman has been fully aroused by clitoral stimulation, she will have difficulty in reaching a climax during intercourse.

- The strength of the orgasm and the ease with which it is reached vary from woman to woman and in the same woman from time to time. Your partner may find she has sensations that are much more intense than usual at certain times of her menstrual cycle or in particular positions.

- Orgasm is not indispensable for a woman's sexual satisfaction. Sometimes, or even always, your partner may feel happy and relaxed after sex without having had one. If this is truly the case, then you need not worry.

- If your partner has had little sex she may not have had an orgasm before. Most women need to learn to experience orgasm as they become more relaxed and confident of their own sexuality.

- Your partner needs continuous stimulation to achieve a climax, and no matter how near she is to it, the pleasurable sensations will die away if you cease to stimulate her.

- Women usually find orgasm easiest to achieve, and often most intense, through masturbation. But many of the women interviewed for the influential Hite report on female sexuality said that even though the intensity of the climax reached this way was greater, they felt a 'vaginal emptiness', a desire to be filled by a penis, which intercourse was better able to satisfy.

- While a man has a 'refractory' period after ejaculation, during which he cannot achieve another erection however much he is stimulated, many women are capable of having another orgasm, and sometimes several more in quick succession, if they are stimulated again shortly after reaching a climax. However, this does not mean that they necessarily want multiple orgasms. Nor does it mean that you have to be a sexual athlete to satisfy your partner. If she wants to have more than one orgasm, you can bring her to her first climax by using your hand or your tongue, and then have intercourse, with or without simultaneous manual stimulation of the clitoris, depending on how aroused she is.

Helping your partner reach orgasm

Clitoral stimulation is the key to orgasm for a woman. If your partner has never experienced a climax, encourage her to masturbate. Almost all women can achieve orgasm through masturbation, and in this way she will learn the most effective methods of stimulating her clitoris. You can then apply these when you make love to her. What is much more likely, however, is that she can climax during masturbation but finds it harder, perhaps even impossible, to do so during intercourse. You will probably find that at least one of the following techniques will make it possible for her. Whichever method you use, make sure that she is highly aroused before you enter her.

Minimum entry

In a man-on-top position, raise yourself on your hands and move just the tip of your penis in and out of her vaginal lips, so that there is a distinct pull on them. This technique will probably not give you the stimulation you seek, but if you employ it between periods of deeper thrusting, it can be very arousing for your partner.

Maximum withdrawal

Withdraw your penis as far as you can after each thrust. This feels very good for most women because it creates the same sensations as the technique described above, pulling the vaginal lips and stimulating the highly sensitive entrance.

Imitating a favorite masturbation method

If your partner usually keeps her legs together when she masturbates, adopt an intercourse position that allows her to do this. If she parts her legs, take up an appropriate position to make her feel equally relaxed (see SEXUAL POSITIONS, p.55).

Dual-stimulation

Choose a position for intercourse in which you can easily reach your partner's clitoris with your hand (see SEXUAL POSITIONS, p.55) so that you can give her additional manual stimulation. Alternatively, suggest that she stimulate herself manually while your penis is inside her.

Alleviating 'performance anxiety'

Like men, women sometimes find that their sexual performance is inhibited by anxiety. It may be that your partner concentrates so much on whether she is pleasing you or is making you impatient because of her failure to come as quickly as she would like to, that she fails to focus on and fully experience her own sensations. Encourage her to forget performance goals and to simply enjoy whatever she feels.

Fear of penetration

Sometimes a woman has such an intense fear of being penetrated or even having her genitals touched that she reacts to every sexual advance by an automatic tightening that is quite beyond her control, of the muscles surrounding her vaginal entrance. This, of course, makes penetration impossible. Often the problem starts after a painful or traumatic experience of intercourse, although it may be the result of a restrictive upbringing that has left her with an irrational fear of sex. Exceptionally, there is a physical reason for this condition, which is known as vaginismus, and so it is always advisable for a woman suffering from it to be examined by a doctor. The condition almost always responds well to loving and patient treatment, so that you can probably help her to overcome it. The following exercise program enlists your help in tackling the problem.

1 Reassure your partner that her fears about her vagina being too small, which is almost certainly how she thinks of it, are the product of her imagination and not based on fact. Explain to her that the vaginal walls are enormously distensible, and that since they can accommodate the passage of a baby, she can take your penis with ease.

2 Encourage her to examine her vaginal area with a mirror, so that she knows exactly how it is formed.

3 This stage will probably be the hardest for her, but once she has managed it, everything else will proceed more smoothly. She should insert just the tip of a well-lubricated finger, as far as the first joint, into her vagina. At first she will probably only feel able to touch the entrance, but it is important that at each attempt she inserts the finger just a little more. When she feels her vaginal muscles tightening, she should pause, deliberately tighten them still more around her finger, and then relax them. After repeating this exercise several times she will begin to feel she has control over her vaginal muscles.

4 When she can fairly comfortably insert one finger as far as it will go into her vagina, she should try using two fingers.

5 She should now feel confident enough to let you insert your finger (after you have checked that you have no jagged fingernails) in the same way. Ask her to relax and tighten her muscles around it.

6 After a few weeks of this exploratory treatment, first with her fingers, then with yours, she should be ready to try intercourse. When you do so, it is important, first, that she is thoroughly aroused (use extra lubrication if necessary) and, secondly, that you let her adopt a woman-on-top position so that she can lower herself onto your penis as slowly and gently as she likes. Do not thrust to begin with, but just let her get used to the sensations caused by the presence of your penis in her vagina.

Throughout this treatment, remember that she is working at overcoming a very profound fear and that it is not to do with her feelings about you but with those about intercourse. Understand that she will be as upset as you are by the reaction of her body, which is completely at odds with the way she wants to react.

Painful intercourse

Sex is rarely painful for a man (see PAINFUL INTERCOURSE, p.35) but there are several conditions, some fairly common, which can cause a woman pain during intercourse. If your partner has such a problem suggest that she see a doctor and wait until the condition has righted itself before you attempt intercourse again.

Painful intercourse is normally due to one or more of the following factors:

☐ Vaginal or bladder infection (by far the most common cause)

☐ An allergy reaction to deodorants, douches, or bath additives

☐ Deep thrusting by the male that aggravates endometriosis (pelvic infection)

☐ Pressure on an ovary owing to retroverted uterus (rare, and painful only in certain positions)

Pain is also common after childbirth, especially if there are episiotomy scars. It may also be the result of a lack of vaginal lubrication, usually either because the woman is insufficiently aroused or because of changes in the vagina due to aging (see below).

Sex and aging

Many women find that their sex drive intensifies in their late thirties and forties. And while the menopause (which usually occurs some time between the ages of 45 and 55) marks the end of a woman's reproductive life, it need not, and seldom does, signal the end of her sexual activity. Sometimes, after the menopause, there is a thinning of the lining of the vagina and a decrease in its lubrication that can make intercourse painful.

If your partner has this problem her doctor may suggest hormone replacement therapy, but lubrication with water or saliva may be all that is needed. It helps too, to keep up an active sex life because this increases the flow of blood to the vagina and helps to retard the effects of aging. Like you, your partner will probably take longer to become aroused as she grows older. Therefore sex is likely to become a more leisurely and relaxed affair, with greater emphasis on the intimacy and comfort of a loving relationship and less on the goal of orgasm.

Conflicting sexual tastes

There are various activities which can be incorporated into an unadventurous sexual routine to provide greater stimulation or variety. If you both enjoy them, they can increase your pleasure as well as strengthening the sexual bond between you. But if one partner dislikes something the other enjoys, or if an activity becomes so important to one of you that it becomes a substitute for your usual sexual activities rather than just enhancing them, you will encounter a conflict of interests. This situation is common, since male and female tastes often diverge widely.

In matters of unconventional or unfamiliar sexual practices there are three cardinal rules:

☐ Do not do it unless you both enjoy it.

☐ Do not do it if it is harmful to either partner.

☐ Do not put pressure on your partner to do it if she clearly does not want to.

Oral and anal sex

Most surveys suggest that fewer women than men include oral sex among their favorite sexual activities. If it is new to your partner, she may be apprehensive when you first suggest it, in part at least because she does not know what is expected of her. You will therefore have to be prepared to give her explicit instructions. Do not expect her to give you oral stimulation unless you are happy to do the same for her. She may or may not want to swallow your semen, and this should be entirely her decision. Do not act as though she is somehow failing you if she prefers not to.

Few women suggest anal sex. Most are convinced that it will hurt or that it is unhygienic, and unless you are very gentle, and wash your penis thoroughly if you are going to have vaginal intercourse afterwards they would be right in each case. There is, in addition, the very real danger that this is an activity which carries a high risk of AIDS. If you are reluctant to give it up because it is something that you and your partner both enjoy very much, wearing a strong condom lubricated with nonoxynol-9 (a substance which destroys the HIV virus) makes it safer. (See **Oral sex**, p.52, **Anal sex**, p.54, and **Guidelines for safer sex**, p.154).

Sadomasochism

The practice of sadomasochism is based on the derivation of sexual pleasure from inflicting and receiving pain. Most sadomasochistic relationships have one dominant and one submissive partner and these roles are often adopted to an extreme degree.

The mildest form of sadomasochism is bondage, in which, in order to heighten the sexual excitement of both, the 'dom' ties or chains the 'sub'. Beating is also a common sadomasochistic practice. Many women go along with mild forms of bondage – if your partner agrees to try it, never tie the neck or head, or subject each other to more pain than the recipient wants – and enjoy gentle fantasy-based games. But if your woman has no real taste for them it is probably because she feels that the situation will get out of hand. She may also find it hard to understand, unless she feels the same way, how loving feelings can be translated into painful or humiliating actions.

Sadomasochistic games are something your partner is more likely to tolerate because you enjoy them rather than because she enjoys them herself. The serious sadomasochist is nearly always male, and the man who has not got a steady partner willing to engage in bondage, flagellation, or similarly motivated practices must turn to prostitutes specializing in these areas.

Fetishism

A mild degree of fetishism – the taste for women in fishnet stockings or fancy underwear, for example – is a feature of most men's sex lives. Fetish objects such as these garments may enhance their sexual excitement but most men are not dependent on them for arousal. However, if you are a true fetishist you will need a special item or set of circumstances in order to become aroused. For example, you will not enjoy sex unless you are wearing rubber. For the extreme fetishist, just wearing rubber, leather, plastic, or fur is all that is needed to produce arousal and orgasm. In such cases the fetish takes over completely and becomes a substitute for a partner.

Fetishism seldom, if ever, occurs in women, so it is unlikely that you will find a partner who truly shares your tastes. You may well find a woman sympathetic to your preferences in this area if they involve her, and she will probably accept that you find it exciting to see her dressed in whatever clothing arouses you. However, it is likely to seriously disturb her if you can only achieve an erection when wearing a particular garment and your sex life will undoubtedly suffer if your fetishism threatens to replace rather than enhance the sex between you.

A few men have a special fetish: they become aroused by dressing in women's clothes. This practice, known as fetishistic transvestism, and the way it may affect your relationship, are examined in more detail in **Transvestism**, p.100.

If you have sexual tastes which your partner finds unacceptable, it may be worth trying to 'shape' these by using fantasies of more acceptable sexual practices during masturbation. You may need to use your usual 'deviant' fantasy to arouse yourself, but then you should deliberately shape the fantasy to follow a 'straight' sexual scenario leading to orgasm. Sadly, some deviations (for example pedophilia) can be so ineradicable and destructive that the only way to alter them is by using drug treatment to reduce all sexual drive.

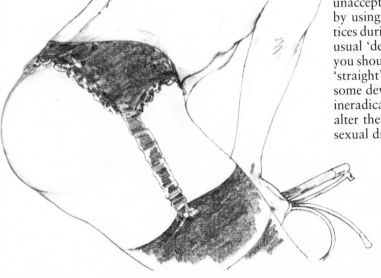

◁ **Power games**
A few people need to act out their fantasy in the form of an elaborate ritual of submission.

AVOIDING SEXUAL BOREDOM

Boredom is seen by many couples as the Catch 22 of their relationship. The argument goes thus: a relationship has more chance of lasting if it is monogamous, but sex with the same partner for 30 years – perhaps more – will inevitably be boring, and boredom, if it does not simply erode the joy from a relationship, may well lead to infidelity and so threaten it even more.

But to assume that sex must eventually become boring without an occasional change of partner, is to underestimate the consolidating and strengthening role that it can play in a long-term relationship and the capacity of a couple to change and adapt.

The inevitability of change

Even though boredom might be avoidable, change is not. The passion and urgency that characterize the first months of a love affair do, eventually, disappear. But for most people this is more than compensated for by the ease and comfort that come from being with a lover whose body has become familiar and whose sexual rhythms have adapted to and accommodated one's own. Long-term lovers know each other's needs and preferences, have discovered what they most enjoy doing together, and accept and trust each other so that anxieties about sexual performance are unnecessary. Such benefits constitute a large part of the reason why many couples still enjoy sex together after many years and why for some it seems to get even better. These things are not possible in a new relationship, however passionate.

Changing attitudes to sex

So why is it that not all established couples experience a strengthening of their sex life together? The first thing to remember is that sexual sensations remain the same; it is only our attitude toward them that changes. The second, if you want to establish the real cause of your boredom, is to look at sex in the wider context of your lives together.

If there is a depressing pall of monotony over everything or if there is so much bad feeling that you do not really enjoy anything you do together, it would be unrealistic to expect sex to be any different. In this case, sexual boredom is only part of a much wider problem. Maybe you need to spend more time together, pay more attention to each other, and have more fun together. After all, that was the reason why

you got together in the first place. Finding a new shared interest, going to see a play or film together, even just passing over to your partner a book you have read and found interesting, will give you points of contact and something interesting to talk about. The busier your lives, the more important it is not to squander the little time you have together. Try to plan your weekends to include activities that you both enjoy. Or 'trade' activities: a concert for her one week, a film for you the next. Seeing each other as more stimulating and interesting may boost your sexual relationship too.

Try to reward each other more, occasionally doing something nice for your partner, not for any particular reason except just to please her. It does not have to be on a grand scale: bringing home flowers, offering to cook the supper if it is usually her job, can induce a feeling that on the whole, life is pleasanter with a partner than without one. Sex will not flourish, it will not even survive unless the basic elements of attraction and affection remain. If your relationship has grown increasingly monotonous, you need to work out what is wrong between you, with the help of professional counselling if need be, so that you can regenerate some of your feelings for each other. Then you can start to revive your sex life.

Combatting sexual boredom

If you are basically happy with the quality of your life together, you have all the more reason for examining the causes of sexual tedium. It is possible that you are bored because sex has become too predictable. If you have developed an unvarying routine, or have a very narrow sexual repertoire, then it is not surprising that a sense of sameness has set in. Try to find more varied ways of sexually arousing each other – a romantic dinner, a game of strip poker or hide and seek.

However, if you are bored in spite of the fact that you have always been sexually innovative and have explored all manner of sexual possibilities, then you probably have a fantasy notion of what sex should be. If so, what you must do is modify your expectations. **Accepting sexual reality**, p. 123, will help you to get the most from the sexual relationship you have.

Breaking your sexual routine

Introducing change into a long-established sexual routine is not easy. After year upon year of the missionary position, to suggest that your partner might like to see what it is like on top may seem to be too revolutionary, either for you to suggest or for your partner to accept. You will both need, first of all, to accept the idea of change, for as long as you both take it for granted that this is the way things are done, they will go on being done that way. Then you should bring about very small or subtle changes in your routine, simply leaving the light on one day, for example, if you usually make love in the dark. EXPANDING YOUR SEXUAL REPERTOIRE, p.48, suggests various changes of this kind and describes positions for intercourse that may be unfamiliar but nevertheless rewarding.

When you discuss such changes with your partner, be careful not to make it seem as though you are criticizing her. The rut you have got into is not exclusively the fault of either of you, since even if you have never suggested varying the routine before, nor has your partner. It is, of course, always the easiest option to accept things as they are. But what you need to do now is to find ways of altering that routine so that it will make sex more fun.

Expressing your needs

Your own fantasies and daydreams are a good way of finding out the kinds of sexual activity you would really like to try. So, too, are past sexual experiences you have particularly enjoyed. It is a good idea to talk to your partner about something in theory before you put it into practice, so that she has time to get used to the idea and perhaps to overcome any inhibitions. This is especially important if what you suggest is unconventional to her.

If you would like your partner to do something for you, one way of indicating this is to do it, or something similar, for her. This kind of non-verbal communication can be very useful if you find it hard to put your sexual wishes into words. But most important of all, if your partner is very resistant to the idea of change, do not press it, at least for the moment. Reassure her that it is because you enjoy sex with her and value the relationship that you want to keep the former as exciting as you can.

Accepting sexual reality

For some people disillusionment occurs because the qualities they valued most in the early stages of a relationship – the passion, excitement, and intensity – tend to fade fastest. Unless you are realistic enough to acknowledge that this is bound to happen, and to learn to value what develops in their place, you may come to regard this calmer, less frenzied phase of the relationship as boring.

It is possible to feel the same sense of dissatisfaction, not because things are not what they used to be, but because reality has failed to meet your expectations. Almost certainly, this is because those expectations are unattainable and your view of sex is a fantasy one. If you continually hanker after ecstasy, you are bound to find simpler pleasures.

Valuing the present

The remedy for entrenched boredom is not to seek new levels of excitement in, for example, fresh sexual activities, an affair, or erotic books or movies. These tactics can add spice when the relationship is a little stale, but only if used in moderation. If they are treated as a last-ditch solution, a fresh process of familiarization will inevitably lead to further disillusionment. Instead, try to feel differently about the way things are right now. It is your attitude toward the present that will determine the degree of your future sexual happiness. Below are some guidelines to getting the best from what is available to you right now.

☐ Examine all the good things about sex with your partner. It may not be as exciting as it once was but at least it is reliable. You can probably judge each other's responses well, and you know the kinds of activity you like best. Also, since you are more relaxed with each other, you can prolong lovemaking much more easily than you could in the excitement of a new relationship.

☐ When you are making love, focus strongly on the physical sensations. These are the same as ever, and if they feel less intense it is probably because you have come to pay less attention to them. To feel the location and intensity of pain more clearly you focus your attention on it. The same principle applies to pleasure.

☐ Live in the here and now: avoid comparisons with past experiences and do not fantasize about those you would like to have in the future.

☐ Do not equate physical affection – the giving of spontaneous hugs or kisses – with sex. They help keep your relationship alive, but need not necessarily indicate that you are making (or expecting) sexual overtures.

☐ You should not forget that a two-way process is involved. You will get feedback from the pleasure you give your partner, for the more she enjoys sex with you, the more she will want to please you.

INFIDELITY

Probably about a quarter to a half of all women have at least one affair during their marriage, and, by the age of 40, two-thirds of married men have been unfaithful. Recent research suggests that these figures may be considerably higher, and also that the 'fidelity gap' between men and women is fast decreasing, perhaps because so many women now go out to work and have the same opportunities as men to meet new partners. It also indicates that women nowadays have their first affair earlier – about four years into the marriage, while men usually become unfaithful after about five years.

However, concern about AIDS and the necessity for safe sex means that casual affairs and 'one night stands' are probably becoming less common. Most affairs are with colleagues and close friends. Men are more likely than women to confess an affair to their partner, maybe because women have more sense, maybe because, some surveys suggest, women are less likely to end a marriage because of a partner's infidelity.

A serious affair nearly always involves a conscious decision, no matter how spontaneous or unexpected you have convinced yourself it is. Think hard before deciding to confess to a liaison. Provided that your infidelity is not symptomatic of any real trouble in your primary relationship, it is your problem, not your partner's.

Why do affairs begin?

If an affair becomes so serious that you begin to think about breaking with your steady partner, it is vital to analyze your reasons for continuing with it if you are not to find yourself in yet another unsatisfactory relationship. Here are some of the main reasons why affairs begin:

☐ *A need for sexual variety or to satisfy curiosity.* Such motivations are especially likely if you have had very few partners. Affairs based mainly on sexual attraction are usually brief and are a poor reason for breaking up your relationship.

☐ *Excitement.* This is the prime reason for some men. The idea of an illicit affair is much more exciting than a legitimate relationship and often a man will ruin a valued relationship through one or more affairs. Sometimes a successful relationship

may seem to present too little challenge, while an affair, with the risks it involves, may make you feel more alive.

☐ *Sexual dissatisfaction with a partner.* An affair may show you what is wrong with sex between you and your partner, and even help you to improve things. But there is a risk that the affair may seem an easier option than working on the problem with your partner, so that you will tend to shelve difficulties rather than solve them.

☐ *To satisfy an emotional need.* The desire to feel loved and wanted in a new way often provides the impetus for entering into an affair.

☐ *To precipitate a crisis in a relationship that is unsatisfactory.* This does not necessarily mean that you want to turn your affair into another permanent relationship. Wait until the heat has died down to see how you really feel.

☐ *As a morale booster.* Sometimes an affair is used to boost self-esteem after a career setback, or as tit-for-tat if it is discovered that a partner has been unfaithful.

☐ *Looking for the perfect lover.* This is the excuse given by the man who maintains that he is really monogamous at heart, if only he could find the perfect mate. Almost certainly, he is fooling himself. If you have always had affairs, the chances are that you will find it hard to change completely. It is easy to avoid commitment, to avoid having to work at a relationship, if you always believe something better will turn up.

The effect on your relationship

Most men believe it is possible to have sex without commitment, and tend to view affairs as something intense but fleeting, that will eventually fade away, leaving their main relationship intact. But however much you want to keep an affair on a casual or friendly basis, emotions can, and often do, get out of hand. An affair is usually embarked upon to meet some unsatisfied need. If it succeeds, it may come to be more and more important to you, affecting your wholehearted commitment to your steady partner, however little you want it to. If she discovers what is going on, it is bound to affect, and may even destroy, your relationship.

For couples who are living together, without being married, the discovery of an affair may be particularly destructive because it will be seen by the injured party as a feasible alternative to their way of life together. The married couple have a built-in stability, practical, financial and social, that makes dissolution much harder and makes it much more likely that they will ride out the storm.

If for whatever reason, you confess to an affair (or are found out) your partner's reaction will depend to a large extent on the length and intensity of that involvement. A casual, brief affair is easier to understand and forgive than one of long duration. In the latter case your partner has to review a substantial section of your life together and come to terms with the fact that the reality of your relationship during this time has been quite different from what she had supposed.

The difficulties of an affair

An affair probably has the best chance of success when it fulfills a simple sexual need for both partners, with no additional demands on either side. But few relationships are as simple as this. Emotional damage to at least one of the parties involved is almost inevitable. Your chances of minimizing this will be improved if you follow a few basic rules:

☐ Learn to compartmentalize your life and your emotions. That is the only way you will be able to give the commitment to each relationship that will enable both to survive.

☐ Do not try to justify what you are doing by focusing on your principal partner's failings.

☐ Do not neglect domestic commitments or let emotional or practical crises build up at home.

☐ Do not spend the necessarily limited time you have with your new lover regretting that it is not more, or bring up when you only have a few more minutes left together tricky issues that cannot easily be resolved. Nearly all affairs have to be managed with one eye on the clock, which may make it difficult to express your feelings spontaneously.

☐ Make sure that the pleasure outweighs the pain brought about by the guilt, the inconvenience, and the often desperate need for secrecy.

☐ If you suspect that your partner is conniving at the affair, making things a little too easy for you, drop it at once if you value her. She may have her own reasons for wanting it to continue, and perhaps you should reexamine your relationship with her more closely to find out just what they are.

Discovering an affair

How to tell if your partner's cheating? Many affairs go undetected for years, but the signs are probably there all the same, at least in the first flush of the affair, when the unfaithful one may seem to be on a constant 'high', though emotionally holding you at arm's length. They may seem more critical or irritable than usual – or suspiciously nicer and more considerate towards you.

Do not seek for confirmation that your partner is having an affair unless you really want to know and you have thoroughly considered all the implications. If it comes to a showdown, remember that the pain of rejection makes the worst possible background against which to conduct a rational discussion that might save your relationship. A bitter and emotional tirade, however justified, precludes any two-way communication and gives your partner no right of reply. There will be details which will seem to you to be of paramount importance at the time: when and where it happened and whether sex was better with the other man, for example.

Planning a solution

Your partner's affair is symptomatic of a need in her. It may be a need you do not recognize or sympathize with, but you will have a better chance of understanding what went wrong if you acknowledge that need. So the first constructive thing you must do is to set aside time to talk about it together, at length and without interruption. At first there are only really two points for discussion: why it happened and how your partner feels now. Your own feelings must be so painfully apparent, so inescapable to both of you, that there is really not much point in laboring them. Scarcely anyone is proof against the hurt that discovery of an affair can cause. But if you want to save the relationship, remember that however you feel, it is in your best interests not to say too much that is unforgivable or unforgettable.

It is important to realize that one instance of infidelity does not mean that your partner has embarked on an endless career of affairs. Many couples survive the discovery of an affair and continue a relationship that will undoubtedly be changed, but may nevertheless be strengthened because of increased mutual understanding.

JEALOUSY

Jealousy is one of the most powerful, destructive, and painful emotions. It is often regarded as a measure of the love one person feels for another. Conversely, the absence of jealousy is often taken as a sign of not caring and an insecure partner may test the other's love by trying to provoke jealousy.

It is more accurate to say that jealousy is a fear of loss rather than a demonstration of love. Unreasonable and frequent jealousy shows not so much that you mistrust your partner but that you cannot trust yourself to hold your relationship together in the face of even the slightest competition. When jealousy runs this deep, the one thing your partner cannot give you is reassurance. Your feelings of insecurity and inferiority are such that you are not prepared to believe anything except the answer that you dread hearing: that there is someone else.

When is jealousy reasonable?
Jealousy is a fear of losing something you value and there are times, when a relationship is threatened, when only a superhuman would fail to feel it. How much jealousy you show is a matter of both judgment and control. The following notes will help you decide whether your (or your partner's) jealousy is justified and will help you handle it.

☐ You are entitled to feel jealous if your partner has been acting suspiciously. If there are sudden significant but unaccountable changes of routine in a partner's hitherto well-organized life, suspicion is probably justified. Suspicion tends to thrive on the accumulation of evidence until it is either substantiated or allayed. It is natural to show flashes of jealousy if your suspicion has been aroused, and to give your partner a warning signal that shows your disquiet.

☐ You are entitled to feel jealous if a partner flirts outrageously with someone else in your presence. This is bad manners on her part and you have a right to complain. She may have had no idea at all that she was hurting you, or she may have been deliberately provoking an outburst because she needs reassurance that you love her, or because she has a grievance that needs airing. Whatever her motives, you can use jealousy positively to force your respective feelings into the open.

☐ Jealousy is unreasonable when it arises solely from your own feelings of inferiority or insecurity. Questioning your partner endlessly about time she spends apart from you because you find it frightening that she has any life outside your relationship is simply destructive and will make her resentful. Searching her handbag or inspecting her belongings for evidence of infidelity is unreasonable, unless you have a solid reason for supposing that she is cheating on you.

☐ Jealousy is unreasonable when it is retrospective. You should not be jealous of people she knew and loved before you were together. The fact that she is with you now should be enough to reassure you of her love. If you are jealous of the past, keep it to yourself.

If you never show your jealousy you are probably very sensible. But do not be so controlled that you fail to take it up with your partner if she is hurting you or jeopardizing your relationship. If you never feel jealous then you are either lucky in being supremely self-confident and absolutely secure in your relationship or you do not care deeply enough about her to mind losing her.

CONTRACEPTION

The fear of an unwanted pregnancy can mar even the best sexual relationship. The pros and cons of the various contraceptive methods available are discussed below, and an indication of their efficiency is also given. Failure rates are given in terms of the percentage of pregnancies that would probably result if 100 healthy young couples used the same method for one year.

It is important to choose a method you are both happy with, and this in itself will help to ensure its success.

The Pill

The contraceptive pill, usually referred to as the Pill, contains synthetic versions of either or both the female hormones estrogen and progesterone. The former prevents ovulation. The latter makes the mucus plugging the entrance to the uterus hostile to sperm and affects the uterus lining, making implantation of a fertilized egg unlikely. The combined pill contains both hormones, and is the most effective. The progesterone-only pill has the fewest side-effects, but is slightly less effective. The 'morning after' pill must be taken within 72 hours of intercourse. Higher in estrogen, it works by expelling the egg, whether fertilized or not.

The side-effects of the Pill vary and a woman may find one brand suits her better than another. But there is unlikely to be a serious risk in taking it, except for women who suffer from, or have a family history of, deep-vein or coronary thrombosis, stroke, or other circulatory disorders, particularly high blood pressure. Doctors also advise women who have diabetes or who are over 35, to change to some other method. Overweight women and smokers are also discouraged from taking the Pill.

Failure rate: less than 1 per cent

The intrauterine device (IUD)

Commonly referred to as an IUD, the intrauterine device is a piece of molded plastic, in some cases containing copper, which is inserted into the uterus. It is second only to the Pill in efficiency, though exactly how it works is still unknown.

An IUD has to be fitted by a doctor or trained nurse, and this will often be carried out during a post-natal visit after pregnancy because insertion is easiest then. The device tends to make a woman's periods longer, heavier and more painful, especially for the first few months after fitting. Because it also seems to render the reproductive system more vulnerable to infection, a woman who has several sexual partners, and so runs an increased risk of contracting a sexually transmitted disease, is probably better off with another form of contraception. The IUD will probably not be recommended for a woman who has not had children but would like to, because if a pelvic infection should develop, infertility can be the result.

Failure rate: 2 per cent

The cap and the diaphragm

These are rubber or plastic devices that fit, in the case of the cervical cap, over the neck of the uterus, or in the case of the diaphragm, across the vagina, to block the passage of sperm. Initially, they must be fitted by a doctor, or other qualified person, and checked each year and after pregnancy. They must be used with a spermicide to be reasonably reliable, and should be kept in place for at least six hours after intercourse. Caps and diaphragms have no disadvantages, apart from the fact that having to insert them before sex may seem to detract from the spontaneity of lovemaking. A very few people are allergic to the rubber of which they are made.

Failure rate: 4 per cent (with spermicide);
15 per cent (alone)

The contraceptive sponge

This device comprises a sponge impregnated with spermicide which is inserted in the vagina before intercourse and left there for a minimum of 24 hours afterward. Like the condom (see below) it is an easily available form of contraception well suited to those with an irregular sex life. However, tests to date on this relatively new product have shown it to be not very competitive with most other contraceptives in terms of efficiency. Therefore it is advisable to use it in conjunction with a condom for greater protection.

Failure rate: up to 25 per cent

The condom (sheath)

The condom is a fine rubber sheath which is rolled onto the erect penis before insertion into the vagina. Care must be taken to expel all the air from the projection at the end before the condom is put on or, if it is of the plain-ended kind, the tip is pinched to deflate it and left free. The ejaculated semen collects in the end of the condom. The base must be held securely during withdrawal after ejaculation to prevent the condom slipping off and releasing the semen. Use a new condom every time you have intercourse. Put it on as soon as erection occurs.

Condoms have always been a valuable method of contraception: they are becoming more popular because they give some protection against AIDS and other sexually transmitted diseases. Some condoms are lubricated with nonoxynol-9, an ingredient of most spermicides, which kills the HIV (AIDS) virus. Use extra spermicide to increase the condom's contraceptive efficiency and give added protection against AIDS if the condom leaks.

Check the date label when you buy condoms (they begin to deteriorate after about two and a half years), and don't expose them to heat or strong light. You will probably need to use additional lubricant, even on those which are ready-lubricated; choose one which is water-soluble, because oil or petroleum-based lubricants will make latex condoms brittle and break easily.

One brand on the market (Mentor contraceptives) has an adhesive inside which seals the condom to the skin, enabling it to stay firmly in place if the penis becomes softer or harder during sex. Scented condoms (to which a few people are allergic) are also available, as are 'ribbed' or textured condoms with a roughened exterior. Some women like the extra stimulation these provide, others find it irritating.

Failure rate: 3 per cent (with spermicide); 15 per cent (alone)

Spermicides

These sperm-killing chemicals are obtainable as creams, jellies, foams, pessaries (gel-coated capsules which are slipped into the vagina) or as squares of impregnated film. They are inserted into the vagina before intercourse, and, because they have only limited efficiency on their own, are normally used in conjunction with a condom, cap or diaphragm. Spermicides containing nonoxynol-9 also kill the HIV virus which causes AIDS.

Failure rate: 25 per cent (alone)

Coitus interruptus (withdrawal)

Withdrawal of the penis before orgasm is the oldest contraceptive method and even now is the most widely used on a global scale. It is among the least efficient of methods, and has only the virtues of being free and always available. The aim of the method is for the man to bring his partner to orgasm through intercourse and then to withdraw the penis and ejaculate outside her. The man who is sexually very competent may be able to use it effectively – some of the time. It is not a good method for someone who lacks good ejaculatory control, or who suffers from 'performance anxiety' (see **Dispelling sexual anxiety**, p.69). Unless you are reasonably relaxed and sexually confident it will be yet another source of worry. Remember that if you have been drinking alcohol or taking drugs, you will have less control than usual. Finally, don't use the method if you have intercourse a second time within a few hours – sperm from the first ejaculation can remain in the pre-ejaculatory fluid.

Failure rate: High

Natural (rhythm) method

Some couples, on religious, moral, health, or esthetic grounds, choose not to use artificial contraceptive techniques. The 'natural' methods they prefer attempt to identify those days around the middle of the menstrual cycle when conception is most likely to occur, and intercourse is avoided at those times. Even so, there are very few absolutely safe days and a couple have to be willing to abstain from sex for a large part of each month if they are to have a reasonable chance of avoiding pregnancy for any length of time.

Natural methods should be practised under the guidance of a doctor or a suitably qualified person. The technique that works best is called the sympto-thermal method. This involves keeping a chart of the woman's early-morning body temperature (which rises slightly just after ovulation) and inspecting the mucus discharge of her vagina (which undergoes certain changes at ovulation). The method has the drawback that it requires a great deal of accurate observation and meticulous record-keeping by the woman. More importantly, if the couple both have a high sex drive they are likely to find it very restricting.

Failure rate: 20 per cent

▽ Choosing a method of contraception

Discuss contraception with your partner and do not assume that it is her sole responsibility. Most methods do in fact demand more of the woman, but this is no reason for her to make the decision alone.

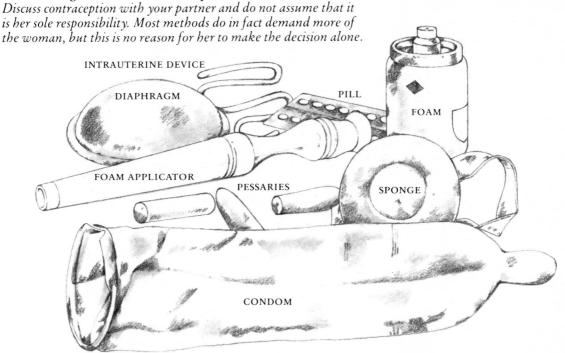

INTRAUTERINE DEVICE

DIAPHRAGM

PILL

FOAM

FOAM APPLICATOR

PESSARIES

SPONGE

CONDOM

VASECTOMY

Both male and female sterilization are totally effective contraceptive techniques and do not affect sex drive. The male operation, known as vasectomy, is a simpler and slightly safer procedure, not even requiring a general anesthetic. Two small incisions are made in the scrotum and the two vas deferens (sperm-carrying tubes) are cut and their ends tied. The whole procedure takes about 20 minutes. Although the tubes can be rejoined, this does not guarantee future fertility, since the semen contains fewer sperm. The operation should therefore be considered irreversible. However, contrary to popular belief, vasectomy does not necessarily reduce sex drive.

The patient is usually advised to wear tight underpants or a jockstrap for a few days after the operation to relieve the dragging feeling in the testes. There may also be some temporary bruising of the scrotum or groin. For about 16 weeks after the operation it is necessary to use additional contraception, since the semen will not be sperm-free until all the sperm present in the vas deferens have been ejaculated. A very few men find that orgasm is painful after a vasectomy.

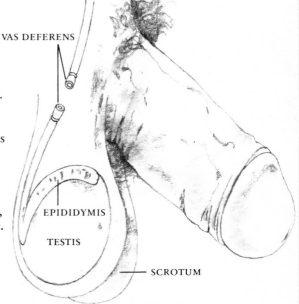

VAS DEFERENS

EPIDIDYMIS

TESTIS

SCROTUM

△ The purpose of vasectomy

Severing and tying the ends of the sperm-carrying tubes prevents sperm from entering the urethra. Consequently, after vasectomy the ejaculate comprises only seminal fluid.

CONCEPTION PROBLEMS

A couple of normal fertility with a typically active sex life – having intercourse two or three times a week – can usually conceive a child within a year. But of every 100 couples, ten are unable to have children and fifteen have fewer than they would like.

A man who is able to have intercourse and to ejaculate usually assumes that because he is potent he must also be fertile, but this is not necessarily so. In some cases of infertility the woman alone is at fault, in some the man, and in some both partners. It is only by microscopic examination that a doctor can tell whether a man's semen is fertile. (None of the notions associating baldness or hairy chests with fertility is true.)

If you have tried for a year and your partner has not been able to conceive, you should visit your doctor together. He will arrange for special tests to be done to establish the cause of infertility, but first he will want confirmation that you have been having sex regularly and that neither of you has a sexual problem (erection difficulties or vaginismus, for example) that makes intercourse difficult. He will then suggest that you concentrate your sexual activity around your partner's most fertile days (two weeks before her period is due). Probably, he will ask whether your partner's periods are regular, for if they are irregular or infrequent the chances of conception are reduced.

Male infertility

By far the most common reasons for male infertility are that the semen either contains too few sperm or too many malformed sperm or that they are not sufficiently mobile. Usually between two and five millilitres of semen are ejaculated at a time, and in order to make conception likely, the concentration of sperm in the semen should probably be more than 60 million per millilitre. If the concentration falls below 20 million per millilitre, the man may well be described as sub-fertile, although conception may still be possible.

Semen infertility is easy to diagnose but difficult to treat, since the precise cause often remains obscure.

Emotional stress, tiredness, and heavy drinking may lower your sperm count temporarily, so it is worth altering your lifestyle if your partner is having difficulty conceiving. Some prescribed drugs also reduce fertility. Your doctor will advise you on this.

Often a few days' abstinence from sex just before your partner's most fertile days may allow a sufficient build-up of sperm to boost your fertility. In some cases drug or hormone treatment can boost sperm production, and occasionally it is possible to collect and concentrate sperm by centrifuging the semen and then, by artificial insemination, introducing it into the woman's uterus. If the problem is a blockage in the sperm ducts, it can be remedied by surgery, but if the semen contains very few sperm or very many abnormal sperm there is little that can be done.

Female infertility

This is more difficult to diagnose, but easier to treat, than male infertility. If tests suggest that your partner seldom ovulates, she may be helped by hormone injections or one of the 'fertility' drugs. Sometimes the problem is a blockage of the fallopian tubes, which carry the egg from ovary to uterus. This can often be cleared by surgery, but if it is not possible, the solution may be *in vitro* fertilization, producing a 'test-tube' baby. In this recently developed and as yet not widely available technique, a ripe egg is taken from the woman's ovary, fertilized with her partner's sperm, and then replaced in the uterus, where it continues normal development.

If you have had sex with your partner for some time and she has not conceived, you may be under considerable stress, not only because of your own desire to have a child, but also because of family and social pressures that are often insensitively brought to bear on the childless couple. Although there is no scientific proof, emotional factors appear to play a part in governing a couple's ability to start a family. Therefore it is worth remembering that the more relaxed you are about the possibility of conception, the greater your chances of success.

SEX AND PREGNANCY

There is no medical reason why intercourse should not continue throughout a normal pregnancy, unless your partner has had a previous miscarriage or she has had a threatened miscarriage during this pregnancy. However, a few men find that the fear of harming the baby during intercourse so inhibits them that they develop erection problems. In fact, the foetus is well cushioned by the uterine fluid and the tightly closed neck of the uterus provides a firm barrier against the outside world.

Maintaining closeness

Often, simply not having to think about contraception, or the relief that conception has taken place if it has been a problem, makes sex during pregnancy even more enjoyable. However, particularly during the first three months, your partner may be less interested in sex than before. The hormonal changes that often make her feel nauseous, tired, or emotional may deprive her of the energy and the inclination for sex, and it may be difficult to arouse her. Avoid intercourse for a while if she feels like this, but do not forget physical intimacy altogether. If she does want to make love, remember that her breasts will be very tender, even in early pregnancy.

Choosing a position

As the pregnancy advances, your partner will find that lovemaking positions that put pressure on her abdomen become increasingly uncomfortable. If you use the man-on-top position, you will need to take more weight than usual on your forearms, and you may find side-by-side, rear-entry, or sitting positions more suitable (see SEXUAL POSITIONS, p.55). A kneeling position may be best if your partner has backache, and is recommended for the final stage of pregnancy because it puts least pressure on the uterus. Indigestion and heartburn may make it uncomfortable for your partner to lie flat on her back, even in early pregnancy, and so she may prefer to make love in a sitting position or at least to prop herself up on pillows.

Sex after childbirth

For a few weeks – usually at least six after a first pregnancy – your partner is likely to feel discomfort, especially if she has had stitches. Her skin may feel tight and prickly even if it seems to have healed, and there may be a very tender area, usually at the base of the vagina, near the anus.

A position in which your partner is on top, or in which you face each other side by side, will avoid putting too much pressure on this sensitive spot. It is best to wait until after her post-natal examination, which should reassure her that everything has returned to normal, before having sex again.

Even if your lovemaking does not include intercourse for the first few weeks, keep up a pattern of loving contact, stimulating each other manually or orally to maintain the flow of physical affection between you, since it is easy to become baby-oriented to the exclusion of each other.

Remember that, even if your partner is breastfeeding, you will need contraception, and the means you were using previously may not be suitable now. Some brands of the Pill are unsuitable at this stage, for example, while your partner will need to be measured for a new diaphragm if you favor this method. (See CONTRACEPTION, p.127.)

Vaginal toning exercises

Childbirth does not, as many men fear, permanently stretch the vagina. The entrance may not be as tight as before, and the muscles may be a little lax, but the postnatal exercises your partner will be advised to do will tone these up. At first it may help to use a position in which your partner's legs are closed, so that your penis is gripped more tightly.

A few women lose interest in sex for a while after they have given birth, usually because tiredness and preoccupation with the baby override all other emotions. Very occasionally this loss of interest is prolonged, and may be a sign of the depression which sometimes occurs after childbirth. In such cases medical treatment is essential.

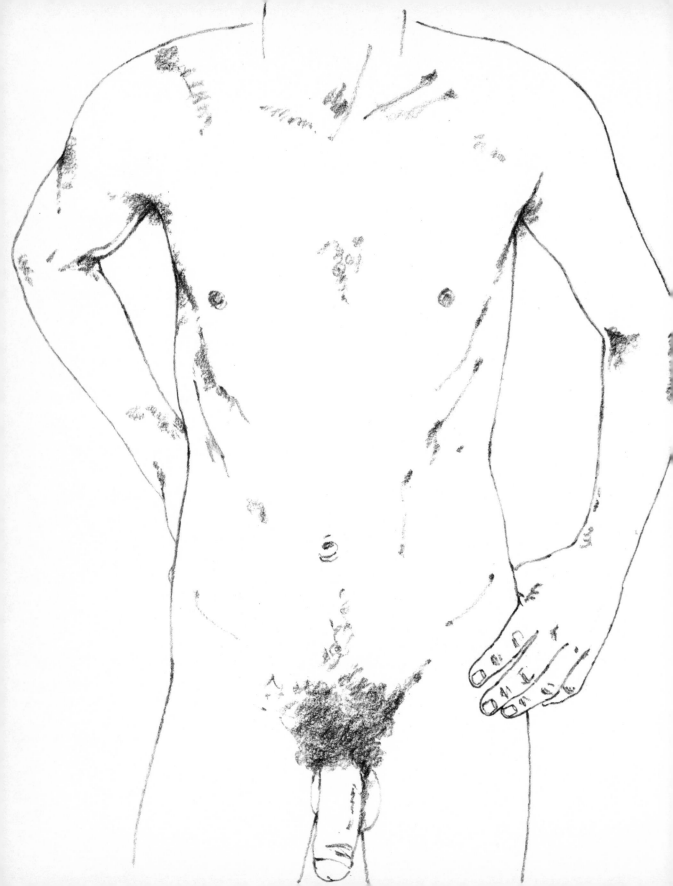

5

THE SINGLE MAN

Some men are single by choice, usually because they do not want to be tied down to a single partner or have not yet found a woman to whom they want to commit themselves fully. Being single is a stage they pass through and enjoy, not a problem requiring immediate solution. However, for many men, being single *is* a problem. While realizing that they would be happier if they could establish a close long-term relationship, they regard commitment and permanence as beyond their grasp.

Among the aims of this part of the book is to widen the single man's options so that if he remains unattached he does so because he wants to, not because he is unable to find a partner or develop a close bond with one woman.

The intention is to make it easier for him to form worthwhile relationships, even if these do not involve a long-term commitment, and to broaden and strengthen the social life on which his sexual contacts will largely depend. The following pages also include advice for the man who is unhappy about being unattached. You may be single because you never seem to meet anyone who might be a potential partner, or because, even when you do meet a woman, you find it hard to start any sort of relationship with her. These difficulties are discussed in the problem chart WHY ARE YOU SINGLE?, p.134. Or your difficulty may lie not in an inability to meet people or to make friends, but in putting a friendly or casual relationship onto a sexual footing. The problem chart DIFFICULTY IN FORMING SEXUAL RELATIONSHIPS, p.138, analyzes some of the reasons for this failure. There are a few men who find that although they have an active sex life, their affairs are always short-lived. Stable relationships elude them and they experience disappointment time after time in their search for permanence. If this is your situation, the problem chart DIFFICULTY IN SUSTAINING RELATIONSHIPS, p.140, will be helpful.

WHY ARE YOU SINGLE?

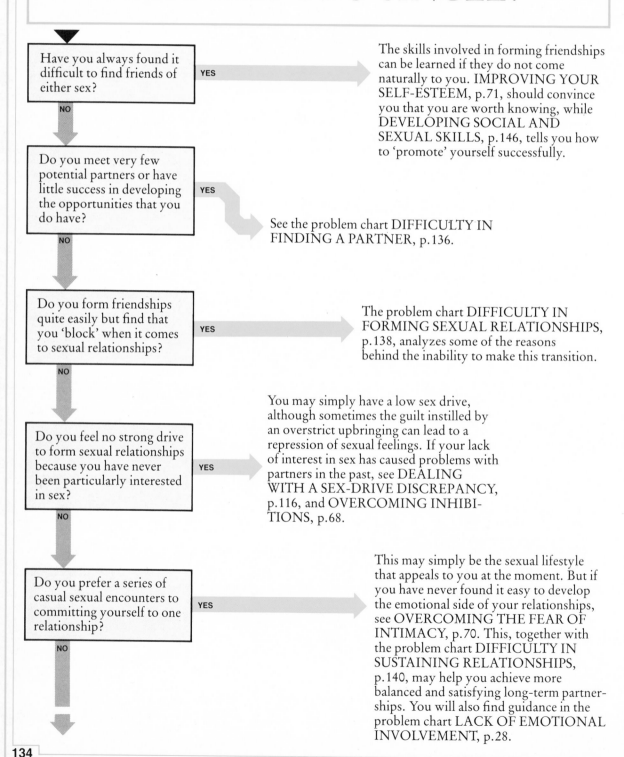

Have you always found it difficult to find friends of either sex?

YES → The skills involved in forming friendships can be learned if they do not come naturally to you. IMPROVING YOUR SELF-ESTEEM, p.71, should convince you that you are worth knowing, while DEVELOPING SOCIAL AND SEXUAL SKILLS, p.146, tells you how to 'promote' yourself successfully.

NO ↓

Do you meet very few potential partners or have little success in developing the opportunities that you do have?

YES → See the problem chart DIFFICULTY IN FINDING A PARTNER, p.136.

NO ↓

Do you form friendships quite easily but find that you 'block' when it comes to sexual relationships?

YES → The problem chart DIFFICULTY IN FORMING SEXUAL RELATIONSHIPS, p.138, analyzes some of the reasons behind the inability to make this transition.

NO ↓

Do you feel no strong drive to form sexual relationships because you have never been particularly interested in sex?

YES → You may simply have a low sex drive, although sometimes the guilt instilled by an overstrict upbringing can lead to a repression of sexual feelings. If your lack of interest in sex has caused problems with partners in the past, see DEALING WITH A SEX-DRIVE DISCREPANCY, p.116, and OVERCOMING INHIBITIONS, p.68.

NO ↓

Do you prefer a series of casual sexual encounters to committing yourself to one relationship?

YES → This may simply be the sexual lifestyle that appeals to you at the moment. But if you have never found it easy to develop the emotional side of your relationships, see OVERCOMING THE FEAR OF INTIMACY, p.70. This, together with the problem chart DIFFICULTY IN SUSTAINING RELATIONSHIPS, p.140, may help you achieve more balanced and satisfying long-term partnerships. You will also find guidance in the problem chart LACK OF EMOTIONAL INVOLVEMENT, p.28.

NO ↓

Do you have a relationship which works well but to which you are hesitant to commit yourself on a long-term basis?

YES → There is no way of guaranteeing a happy-ever-after partnership. But **Factors which make a relationship work or fail**, p.145, indicates the main pointers to success or failure, so that you can at least establish the odds.

NO

Do your relationships usually start well but end disastrously time after time?

YES → If your relationships never last, it may be that you are not choosing well, or that you are not yet clear about the things that matter most to you. Consult the problem chart DIFFICULTY IN SUSTAINING RELATIONSHIPS, p.140.

NO

Do you have a very clear image of the kind of partner you want, so that you 'screen' women you meet almost entirely by their looks, and do few of them measure up to this ideal?

YES → The more rigid your blueprint for a prospective partner, the less likely it is that you will find a woman to match it. WHAT KIND OF PARTNER ARE YOU LOOKING FOR?, p.142, should enable you to see whether you are limiting your options by being inflexible.

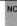

NO

Do you find that most of the women you are attracted to are involved with someone else?

YES → If this happens often it suggests that you do not want to get involved just yet. This tactic provides the safest way of looking as though you are trying while ensuring that you do not succeed. It also points to a reluctance to let yourself become emotionally close to people. You will need to overcome this reserve if you are to make a lasting relationship. See OVERCOMING THE FEAR OF INTIMACY, p.70.

NO → You are probably single because at the moment it suits you. Perhaps it is because you want a break from relationships or because you are giving so much of your time and energy to something else – work, for example – that you cannot make a full-time commitment. Solitude can become a habit though, so if you want eventually to share your life with someone, try not to remain detached from close relationships for long.

CELIBACY

Many men go through periods when for various reasons they need to be alone or free from sexual involvement. Such periods of abstinence can often prove beneficial to you, and you may find that you miss the warmth and the closeness of a partner more than sex. However, self-imposed abstinence of longer than a few months suggests that there is another reason for your lack of interest in sex (see problem chart LACK OF INTEREST, p.24) or that you are using celibacy to opt out of close relationships (see problem chart LACK OF EMOTIONAL INVOLVEMENT, p.28).

MEN ♂ 5 THE SINGLE MAN

DIFFICULTY IN FINDING
A PARTNER

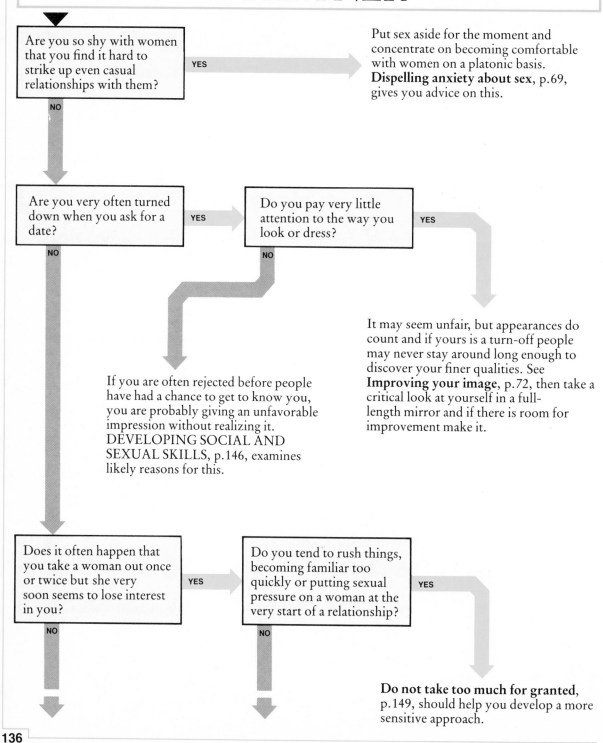

Are you so shy with women that you find it hard to strike up even casual relationships with them?

YES → Put sex aside for the moment and concentrate on becoming comfortable with women on a platonic basis. **Dispelling anxiety about sex**, p.69, gives you advice on this.

NO ↓

Are you very often turned down when you ask for a date?

YES → Do you pay very little attention to the way you look or dress?

YES → It may seem unfair, but appearances do count and if yours is a turn-off people may never stay around long enough to discover your finer qualities. See **Improving your image**, p.72, then take a critical look at yourself in a full-length mirror and if there is room for improvement make it.

NO ↓

If you are often rejected before people have had a chance to get to know you, you are probably giving an unfavorable impression without realizing it. DEVELOPING SOCIAL AND SEXUAL SKILLS, p.146, examines likely reasons for this.

NO ↓

Does it often happen that you take a woman out once or twice but she very soon seems to lose interest in you?

YES → Do you tend to rush things, becoming familiar too quickly or putting sexual pressure on a woman at the very start of a relationship?

YES → **Do not take too much for granted**, p.149, should help you develop a more sensitive approach.

NO ↓

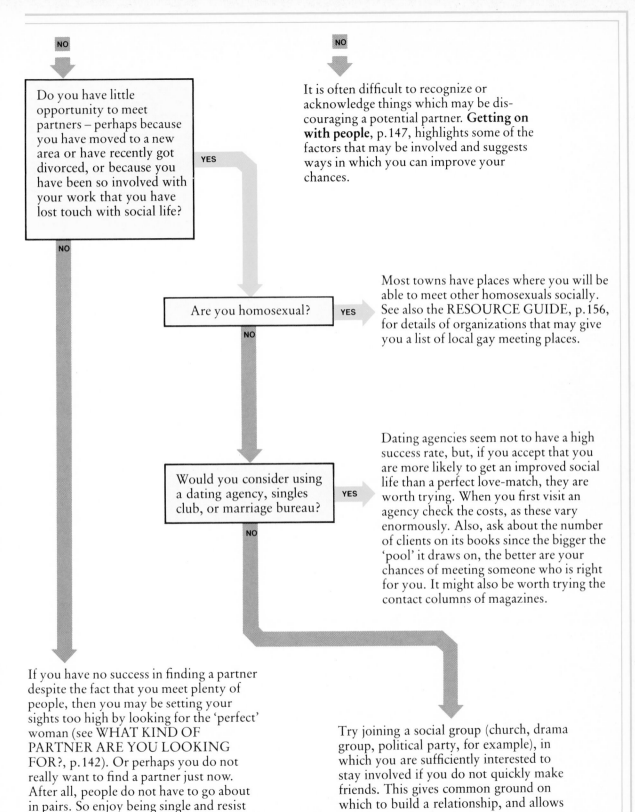

Do you have little opportunity to meet partners – perhaps because you have moved to a new area or have recently got divorced, or because you have been so involved with your work that you have lost touch with social life?

YES

NO

It is often difficult to recognize or acknowledge things which may be discouraging a potential partner. **Getting on with people**, p.147, highlights some of the factors that may be involved and suggests ways in which you can improve your chances.

Are you homosexual?

YES

NO

Most towns have places where you will be able to meet other homosexuals socially. See also the RESOURCE GUIDE, p.156, for details of organizations that may give you a list of local gay meeting places.

Would you consider using a dating agency, singles club, or marriage bureau?

YES

NO

Dating agencies seem not to have a high success rate, but, if you accept that you are more likely to get an improved social life than a perfect love-match, they are worth trying. When you first visit an agency check the costs, as these vary enormously. Also, ask about the number of clients on its books since the bigger the 'pool' it draws on, the better are your chances of meeting someone who is right for you. It might also be worth trying the contact columns of magazines.

If you have no success in finding a partner despite the fact that you meet plenty of people, then you may be setting your sights too high by looking for the 'perfect' woman (see WHAT KIND OF PARTNER ARE YOU LOOKING FOR?, p.142). Or perhaps you do not really want to find a partner just now. After all, people do not have to go about in pairs. So enjoy being single and resist pressure to become part of a couple.

Try joining a social group (church, drama group, political party, for example), in which you are sufficiently interested to stay involved if you do not quickly make friends. This gives common ground on which to build a relationship, and allows you time to develop it at your own pace.

DIFFICULTY IN FORMING SEXUAL RELATIONSHIPS

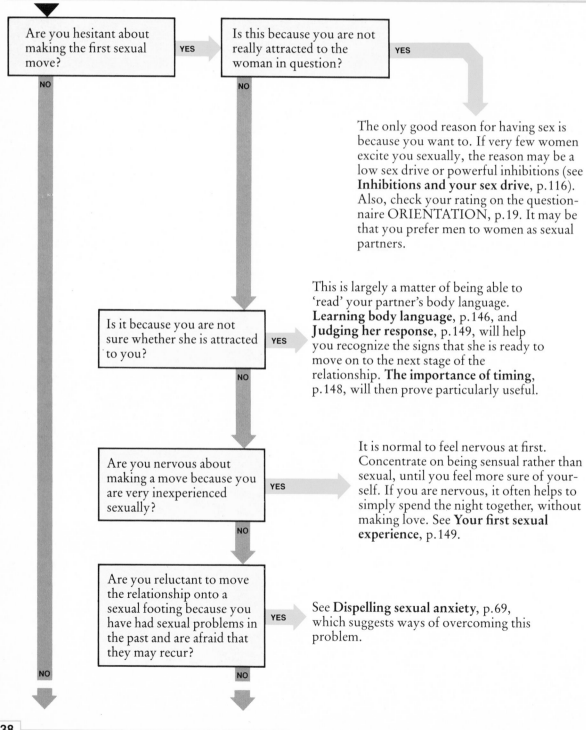

Are you hesitant about making the first sexual move?

YES → **Is this because you are not really attracted to the woman in question?**

YES → The only good reason for having sex is because you want to. If very few women excite you sexually, the reason may be a low sex drive or powerful inhibitions (see **Inhibitions and your sex drive**, p.116). Also, check your rating on the questionnaire ORIENTATION, p.19. It may be that you prefer men to women as sexual partners.

NO ↓ **Is it because you are not sure whether she is attracted to you?**

YES → This is largely a matter of being able to 'read' your partner's body language. **Learning body language**, p.146, and **Judging her response**, p.149, will help you recognize the signs that she is ready to move on to the next stage of the relationship. **The importance of timing**, p.148, will then prove particularly useful.

NO ↓ **Are you nervous about making a move because you are very inexperienced sexually?**

YES → It is normal to feel nervous at first. Concentrate on being sensual rather than sexual, until you feel more sure of yourself. If you are nervous, it often helps to simply spend the night together, without making love. See **Your first sexual experience**, p.149.

NO ↓ **Are you reluctant to move the relationship onto a sexual footing because you have had sexual problems in the past and are afraid that they may recur?**

YES → See **Dispelling sexual anxiety**, p.69, which suggests ways of overcoming this problem.

NO ↓

NO ↓

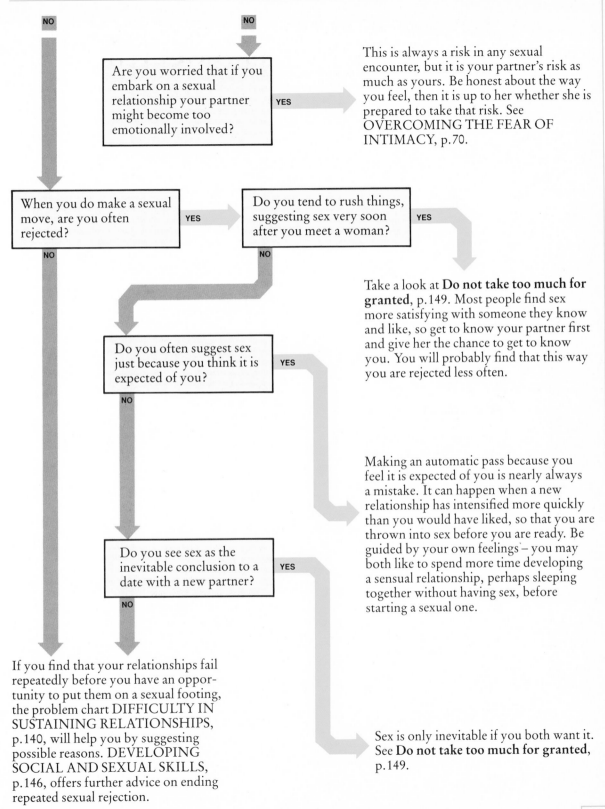

Are you worried that if you embark on a sexual relationship your partner might become too emotionally involved?

YES → This is always a risk in any sexual encounter, but it is your partner's risk as much as yours. Be honest about the way you feel, then it is up to her whether she is prepared to take that risk. See OVERCOMING THE FEAR OF INTIMACY, p.70.

When you do make a sexual move, are you often rejected?

YES → Do you tend to rush things, suggesting sex very soon after you meet a woman?

YES ↓

Take a look at **Do not take too much for granted**, p.149. Most people find sex more satisfying with someone they know and like, so get to know your partner first and give her the chance to get to know you. You will probably find that this way you are rejected less often.

Do you often suggest sex just because you think it is expected of you?

YES →

Making an automatic pass because you feel it is expected of you is nearly always a mistake. It can happen when a new relationship has intensified more quickly than you would have liked, so that you are thrown into sex before you are ready. Be guided by your own feelings – you may both like to spend more time developing a sensual relationship, perhaps sleeping together without having sex, before starting a sexual one.

Do you see sex as the inevitable conclusion to a date with a new partner?

YES →

If you find that your relationships fail repeatedly before you have an opportunity to put them on a sexual footing, the problem chart DIFFICULTY IN SUSTAINING RELATIONSHIPS, p.140, will help you by suggesting possible reasons. DEVELOPING SOCIAL AND SEXUAL SKILLS, p.146, offers further advice on ending repeated sexual rejection.

Sex is only inevitable if you both want it. See **Do not take too much for granted**, p.149.

MEN ♂ **5** THE SINGLE MAN

DIFFICULTY IN SUSTAINING RELATIONSHIPS

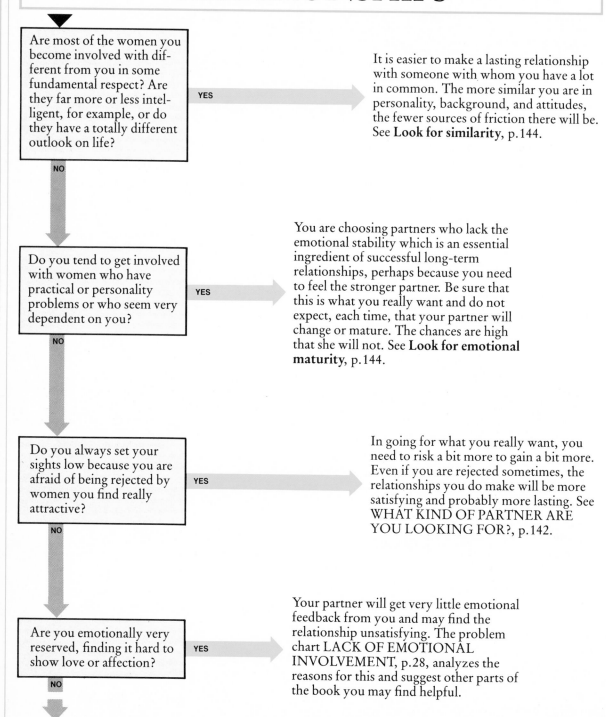

Are most of the women you become involved with different from you in some fundamental respect? Are they far more or less intelligent, for example, or do they have a totally different outlook on life?

YES → It is easier to make a lasting relationship with someone with whom you have a lot in common. The more similar you are in personality, background, and attitudes, the fewer sources of friction there will be. See **Look for similarity**, p.144.

NO

Do you tend to get involved with women who have practical or personality problems or who seem very dependent on you?

YES → You are choosing partners who lack the emotional stability which is an essential ingredient of successful long-term relationships, perhaps because you need to feel the stronger partner. Be sure that this is what you really want and do not expect, each time, that your partner will change or mature. The chances are high that she will not. See **Look for emotional maturity**, p.144.

NO

Do you always set your sights low because you are afraid of being rejected by women you find really attractive?

YES → In going for what you really want, you need to risk a bit more to gain a bit more. Even if you are rejected sometimes, the relationships you do make will be more satisfying and probably more lasting. See WHAT KIND OF PARTNER ARE YOU LOOKING FOR?, p.142.

NO

Are you emotionally very reserved, finding it hard to show love or affection?

YES → Your partner will get very little emotional feedback from you and may find the relationship unsatisfying. The problem chart LACK OF EMOTIONAL INVOLVEMENT, p.28, analyzes the reasons for this and suggest other parts of the book you may find helpful.

NO

Are the emotional ties between you and your parents very strong and is it important for you to have their support and approval in everything you do?

YES ➤ Unless you can achieve real emotional independence, your adult relationships will always be at risk. See **Learning to be more assertive**, p.73, for advice on how to become more independent.

NO

Do you get very jealous of anyone your partner shows even a slight interest in or liking for?

YES ➤ Your relationships might last longer if you had more confidence in your own ability to sustain them. IMPROVING YOUR SELF-ESTEEM, p.71, should help you to achieve this.

NO

Do you feel that whatever goes wrong in your relationships must be your fault?

YES

NO

Are you very moody or inclined to lose your temper easily?

YES ➤ Anger is one of the most destructive elements in any relationship. **Dealing with anger**, p.115, discusses ways of expressing this feeling that will not hurt or alienate your partner irretrievably.

NO

Do you find that although you are very attracted to a partner at first, you lose interest as soon as the relationship shows signs of becoming serious?

YES ➤ This reluctance to commit yourself may be because you fear a close relationship. See OVERCOMING THE FEAR OF INTIMACY, p.70, which analyzes some of the reasons for this and directs you to parts of the book that may be helpful.

NO

If you are still uncertain about why your relationships tend to fail, see **Factors which make a relationship work or fail**, p.145. This suggests other factors to consider if you are starting a relationship which you hope will last.

MEN ♂ **5** THE SINGLE MAN

WHAT KIND OF PARTNER ARE YOU LOOKING FOR?

For some men, sexual interest is so easily awakened that they are attracted to any number of women, and it is not a problem to find a desirable partner. By complete contrast, a few spend years searching for their ideal woman with the same success as if they were questing for the unicorn.

Looks are of paramount importance in sexual attraction for some men, while for others personality is more crucial. For most, though, sexual interest is stimulated by a partner's physical appearance and will then either intensify or die away as her personality reveals itself. Accordingly, you probably have your physical preferences – blondes rather than brunettes, for example, or rounded women rather than angular ones. You may even have a mental image of your ideal partner, but even if, on rare occasions, reality and imagination have a transitory meeting, you cannot expect this to happen often. What is much more common is that you find yourself attracted to someone who bears only a passing resemblance to your perfect woman.

The dangers of inflexibility

Problems may arise, however, when you have such strong ideas about what your partner should be like that you cannot feel attracted to someone who does not conform to them. Obviously, the more rigid your requirements, the less chance there is of finding someone to suit you. Inflexibility is a disadvantage in a long-term relationship too. People change, and your partner will grow older, possibly fatter, certainly grayer. If this matters a great deal to you it may endanger the relationship. The personality too is subject to change, and this becomes particularly apparent if you were both young when you met and have matured together.

The danger in holding out for the perfect partner, quite apart from the fact that she probably does not exist, is that it will prevent you from making the most of the relationships you do have. You may never feel able to make a proper commitment and put everything into a relationship if you are perpetually hoping that something better will come along.

ASSESSING YOUR FLEXIBILITY

The following set of exercises will help you judge whether you are limiting yourself and your sexual opportunities by being too rigid and demanding in your preferences.

1 PHYSICAL PREFERENCES

The aim of the first exercise is to discover which physical characteristics influence your choice of a partner, and how important they are to you.

1 Make a list of ten women you consider physically attractive. They need not be women you know well, or feel a strong sexual attraction to, but simply females whose looks you admire.

2 Next make a list of ten women you do not consider attractive. (Remember, all you are concerned with in these two lists is physical appearance.)

3 Now try to find one quality you really like about each of the women in the first list. List these preferred qualities under the heading 'Positive'.

Then, returning to the list of women you find unattractive, compile a list under the heading 'Negative' of ten physical attributes that you see as unattractive in those women. It may occur that you include the opposite of a quality you write down in the preceding list: 'fat', for example, in the second list, while you put 'slim' in the list of positive attributes. This does not matter.

4 Work through the lists of positive and negative attributes carefully, deciding how important each attribute is to you. Put a mark beside those which, in either a positive or a negative way, are essential to your sexual interest. For example, if one of your preferences is height, put a mark beside that, while if red hair is such a turn-off for you that you could never feel attracted to a redhead, mark that characteristic. Do not mark attributes that you consider important but not indispensable.

Now go on to the second exercise, in which you are asked to apply a similar vetting procedure to personality traits.

2 PERSONALITY PREFERENCES

Even when you meet someone you think looks attractive, she does not necessarily excite you sexually. Nearly always it is some personality trait that tips the balance. You can analyze which of these 'turn-ons' and 'turn-offs' are important to you just as you did previously with physical attributes.

1 Think of the women you know reasonably well and consider to be physically attractive.

2 Now, of these women, select and list ten who arouse you sexually, or have done at some time, and then in a second list ten who, despite their looks, have never excited any real sexual feelings in you.

3 Next, find ten personality traits among the first ten women that you consider attractive and list these under all the heading 'Positive'. Then list ten unattractive personal characteristics that you find in the second group, listing these under 'Negative'.

4 Decide which of these positive and negative traits are so important as to be indispensable to your sexual interest and put a mark beside them.

Your lists of attractive and unattractive qualities, both physical and personal, constitute your own blueprint for sexual attraction. These qualities are what is needed (though not, of course, *all* that is needed) if you are to be sexually attracted to a woman. The number of marks you have put down indicates how rigid this blueprint is. Even one or two emphasized preferences on each list implies that you are to some extent limiting your choice of potential partners. Most men can feel attracted to a woman provided she satisfies at least some of their 'turn-on' requirements, and as long as these outweigh the 'turn-offs' there will probably be at least some sexual interest. The fewer marks there are, the more flexible you are and the more women you will find suitable as prospective sexual partners.

Making yourself more flexible

If your blueprint is very inflexible, it is probably worth trying to change your expectations. The best way to do this is to concentrate your attention on the things about your present partner (or a woman you are currently interested in) that do appeal to you. You will probably find that these are qualities that you have listed in the preceding exercises as important but not vital to your sexual interest. You will probably be able to discover additional qualities you may not have listed as important but which seem special in this person. It is a question of focusing on the positive aspects and of turning your attention back to them when it wanders off.

An alternative is to try to modify your partner so that she fits your blueprint. A tactful man may suggest some change of hair color or style, or diet, but change is not always possible and even if it is, your partner may be happy as she is. If you want to try this, the only fair way is to propose a trade-off. Therefore be prepared to do what you can to alter your own appearance so that it fits your partner's sexual blueprint (which she too may want to check by modifying the above method) more accurately.

Meeting a partner's needs

Once you have found your ideal partner, what then? A few months or years into a relationship, the disillusioned cry is often: 'We were so in love once, why can't it be like that now?' It is unrealistic to expect to keep or recapture the heady feeling of being 'in love'. But that does not mean that an idyllic affair has to become either humdrum or hostile. Behaviour and feelings are closely linked; when behaviour changes, a change in feelings will usually follow. By changing your behaviour you will usually spark off a change in your partner's behaviour too.

A relationship works best when both partners satisfy most of each other's needs for much of the time. So it is important to identify these needs, and to be able to communicate them to each other. See LEARNING TO COMMUNICATE, p.114.

Show appreciation

Carrots are better than sticks if you want to alter another person's behaviour, whether it is a child, a colleague or a sexual partner. So use compliments to show your appreciation when your partner does something that makes you happy, and try to avoid blaming or criticizing them when things go wrong.

MAKING A LASTING RELATIONSHIP

It is difficult to predict the chances of success of any relationship, for the most unlikely partnerships survive for years, while others collapse which seem to have everything in their favor. Nevertheless, the observations of marriage guidance counselors and studies of the causes of marital breakdown suggest that certain factors predispose a relationship to either success or failure. If you are wondering about your chances of making a lasting partnership, below are some of the most important factors to consider.

☐ *Do not commit yourself too young.* Youthful marriages run the greatest risks of all. Every major study of marriage shows that commitments made before the age of 19 are the least likely to survive (especially if embarked upon because the woman is pregnant). As you mature, you will change, developing different needs and interests from one another. It is possible for two people to move in more or less the same direction, continuing to meet each other's changing needs, but far more likely that you will grow apart.

☐ *Do not commit yourself too soon.* You should not consider making a relationship permanent until you have known each other for at least nine months. It takes most people that long to get to know the best and worst of each other, and living with someone is the best way to discover whether your partnership is likely to stand the test of time. A stormy involvement is a danger sign. If you have frequent quarrels and, even worse, if one or other has broken off the relationship more than once, it augurs badly for the future, for the pattern is one that is likely to become established. Protracted dating can be suspect too. If you have been talking about, but postponed, a permanent relationship for a couple of years or more, look carefully at your motives. It may be that you are not yet really ready to lose your independence.

☐ *Look for similarity.* Studies have shown that there is a tendency for people of similar disposition to marry. While some marriages of opposites do succeed, living together without friction is obviously easier for the couple who have similar interests and attitudes and want much the same things from life. It helps to have at least one or two major interests in common and it is probably best to be similar in age as well. If there is a difference of more than ten years between you, it is likely that there will be differences in outlook that are too great for an easy relationship to develop.

☐ *Look for sexual compatibility.* Sex will not prove the binding force it can be if your attitudes toward it are very different, or if it plays a much more (or much less) important part in your life than it does in your partner's. Sexual compatibility is not a matter of technique, and the mechanics of successful lovemaking can be learned as a couple adjust to each other. But it is important that you are truly attracted to and aroused by each other, for it is only on this basis that you will be able to accommodate each other's sexual needs. Given a background of mutual attraction and love, nearly all sexual problems are soluble; without it most are likely to prove insurmountable.

☐ *Look for emotional maturity.* Some personality traits seem to bode particularly ill for the future of a long-term relationship. Frequent expressions of anger, whether they are in the form of rages, the desire to dominate, or a tendency to be hypercritical, are the worst danger sign. And while a relationship may just be able to survive with one partner who feels like this, two will almost certainly doom it to failure. Low self-esteem also signals trouble, as it produces the insecurity and jealousy that will make a loving and trusting relationship hard to attain.

Overdependence can make an adult and lasting relationship impossible. A partner who is still very reliant on parental support and approval may demand more reassurance from you than you have time or, indeed, are prepared, to give. And on the inevitable occasions when you are the one who needs, if only temporarily, to be dependent and supported, she may be quite unable to take the responsibility.

☐ *Make sure that your partner can provide physical closeness and affection.* A person who is emotionally isolated and finds it hard to show affection or to accept it, has poor prospects of sustaining a fulfilling relationship.

□ *Look for flexibility.* The ability to adapt to change is one of the most important attributes to look for in a partner. Neither individuals nor partnerships are static, and a person who is uncompromising may find it hard to meet the changing needs and circumstances of a long-term relationship. It is a good sign if, for example, she is willing to think about new ideas or try new activities, or can adapt easily to last-minute or altered plans.

□ *Do not expect your partner to change.* If you have serious doubts about the relationship, forget it. It is a mistake to enter an unpromising relationship in the hope that your partner will change. If you can live with her as she is now, fine. But if you find yourself hoping that she will become, under your own moderating influence, less moody or extravagant, slower to anger, or less prone to jealousy, you are running a considerable risk. Some people have a great capacity for change, others are the opposite. So if the change matters to you, look for signs of it before you commit yourself, not after.

One ingredient essential for success is not listed above because it requires special emphasis. This is your own certainty about the relationship and the resultant determination to make it work. If you have reservations about your partner, they are likely to grow, and will prevent you from giving the relationship the 100 per cent commitment which more than anything will help it to overcome problems and survive.

Use the chart below to assess the chances of your relationship. In the column on the left are the bonus factors that are likely to increase your chances of success. These do not guarantee bliss, of course, but they do mean that you are likely to have a more contented life together. In the right-hand column are the risk factors. It seems easier to predict disaster than contentment, partly at least because it attracts more attention: more research has been carried out into the reasons for the break-up of relationships than into the factors which help couples to stay happily together. So it is more a cause for concern if you check several items on the 'risk' list than if you fail to check many bonus items.

FACTORS WHICH MAKE A RELATIONSHIP WORK OR FAIL

BONUS FACTORS		RISK FACTORS	
□ Successful cohabitation for at least six months	□ Emotional stability	□ Marrying too young (before 19 years of age)	□ Anger
□ Similar educational and social backgrounds	□ Similar need and enthusiasm for sex	□ Premarital pregnancy	□ Emotional coldness
□ Similar intelligence	□ Flexibility and adaptability	□ Marrying to escape an unhappy home	□ Poor self-image – reflected in low self-confidence
□ Less than ten years difference in age	□ Emotional self-sufficiency	□ Marrying 'on the rebound'	□ Fear of independence
□ Similar attitudes on major issues	□ Ability to give and receive affection	□ Short involvement (under nine months)	□ Possessiveness or extreme jealousy
□ Shared interests and activities	□ Consideration for others	□ Frequent friction or break-ups	□ Selfishness or self-centeredness
□ Similar ambitions and enjoyment of similar lifestyle	□ Similar physical attractiveness	□ Emotional instability	□ Substantial difference in physical attractiveness

DEVELOPING SOCIAL AND SEXUAL SKILLS

The term 'social skill' simply means the art of getting along with people, making them feel by what you say and the way you behave that you like them – and that you are likeable too. Your social skill determines how well you carry off a first meeting, how easy you find it to make friends, and how smoothly you manage to make the transition from a social to a sexual relationship. The handling of this last situation calls for another set of skills, which we shall examine after looking at ways in which you can acquire an easy social manner.

Learning body language

Much of the time, especially at the beginning of a relationship, words are too crude a tool to convey the subtle shades of feeling passing between two people. When you scarcely know each other, the messages 'I like you', 'I'd like to get to know you better', 'Let's take this a stage further' are largely conveyed by body language, a system of communication based on the way you stand, move, and look at each other. You will both respond to this, although you may be unaware of doing so.

A natural body language is something we are born with, but shyness or lack of self-confidence can often make us suppress these natural responses. Shy people, for example, often unwittingly send out the wrong signals, so that their shyness is misinterpreted as boredom, lack of interest, or even hostility. If you can learn to overcome your self-consciousness and increase your self-esteem (see p.71–3), you will be able to respond to people in a more relaxed and natural way.

Eye contact

Always look at the person you are talking to, not over her shoulder (which suggests that you are bored or inattentive) or down at the floor (which indicates that you are shy or even shifty). If she drops her eyes you are probably holding your own gaze for rather too long. What most people find comfortable is intermittent eye contact, for about five seconds in every half minute. This shows that you are interested but not putting the other person under uncomfortably close scrutiny.

When you are sexually interested in a woman, eye contact is one of the simplest and most unmistakable ways of showing it. Hold your glance longer than you would in an ordinary social situation, but again, do not overdo it. You will be able to judge her feelings by the way she responds. If she returns your gaze steadily, this could be an indication of her own interest. If she drops her eyes or shifts her gaze away it could mean that she is not interested, although it may simply be a sign that she is shy and that you are moving too fast. Watch movies or television if you want to see how it is done, for successful actors have long relied on the sustained, smouldering look to express interest in the opposite sex.

Facial expression

It is all too true that you are usually taken at face value. If you look miserable or worried, people will assume that this is the way you feel. If you are often asked if you are feeling OK or are worried about something when in fact you are fine, then your face is not giving the message you want to convey. Smiling is especially important for it is the most direct way of telling a woman that you like her, or that you find her attractive. At the very least, it makes you look friendly and responsive and opens up the possibility of greater closeness.

Gestures

Use your hands to add emphasis and interest to what you are saying. This is something that is often easiest to learn by watching others. There is no need to be dramatic as quite small movements are usually all that is necessary. Head movements are important when you are listening because they encourage the other person to continue speaking as well as indicating your own interest.

Posture

You will give an impression of self-confidence – however you feel – if you stand straight and hold your head up. When you first meet someone, it is best not to stand either too close or too far away. Many people feel uneasy if a stranger stands right next to them since it seems like an invasion of their personal space. On the other hand, physical proximity is a sign of attraction and it is one of the cues you can give when you want to advance a relationship and put it on a more intimate footing. By contrast, standing much farther away often gives an impression of aloofness or even mistrust.

Touching

Use a discreet touch as another signal that you find a woman attractive. Watch carefully for the response you get so that you do not overstep the line between showing interest, which is usually welcome, and 'pawing', which is not. Gentle pressure on a woman's hand or arm as you greet her or say goodbye, for example, is more affectionate and less formal than a handshake, but less intimate than a kiss. Once you have established contact you can step up the relationship by more prolonged or more frequent touching. Move from 'safe' gestures – a brief touch on her knee to emphasize a point as you are talking, brushing her hand with your own as you pass her something, holding it for a moment or two as you say goodbye – to more overtly sexual ones. Hold her hand in the cinema or as you walk down the street. If she does not draw away, and especially if she is starting to make the same gestures to you, the chances are that you will soon be able to move to the next stage, the hugging and kissing that lead to exploration and caressing of each other's bodies.

Listen to your voice

Your voice, after your appearance, makes the strongest initial impact on the people you meet. You can get an impression of how others hear you by listening to a tape recording of yourself. Few people like the sound of their own voice at first, but try to pick out the characteristics that might make it difficult or irritating for others to listen to and that you may be able to modify. Do you mumble, for example? Resolve to speak more clearly and loudly enough to be heard easily without creating a harsh effect. Does your voice sound high-pitched or monotonous? Try to lower it a little or to vary the tone. Put expression into your speech, but do not overemphasize individual words. Conversation, not oratory, is what you need to become proficient in. Try also to identify and eliminate irritating mannerisms such as frequent hesitation or nervous giggles.

Getting on with people

Conversation is the prime ingredient of social success. If you can handle it well, you will make a good first impression on people you meet and it will carry you with confidence through the opening stages of a new relationship. If you find it hard to talk to people, or if they seem unresponsive to you or seldom follow up the first encounter, it is possible that you have unwittingly developed some bad conversational habits. The following notes will help you if this is the case.

☐ Keep the conversation fairly neutral at first, so that either of you can back off easily if you want to. Talk about things which could not possibly offend or lead to heart-searching before moving on to more personal matters. It is a mistake to tell too much too soon. If you embark on an immediate outpouring of the intimate details of your personal life you will frighten off the other person with your intensity.

☐ Do not, when you first meet someone, either undersell or oversell yourself. It is normal to try to present yourself in a flattering light, but remember that a false image may be difficult to live up to (or hard to live down).

☐ Do not wander off the point of conversation, talk too much about yourself, or interrupt continually when someone else is talking.

☐ Never answer a question with a flat yes or no. This ends a conversation as soon as it has started. Expand your answer somehow, giving the other person a cue to continue the discussion.

☐ Talk about what really interests you and be positive in what you say. It is even better if you can find something you have in common – a shared interest or a mutual friend – to get the conversation going.

☐ Try not to let lengthy pauses develop. If you cannot think of a new topic, follow up what the other person last said with a comment or, preferably, a question that renews the discussion.

☐ When you are listening, remember that this is not a totally passive role. Every now and then make some encouraging response to stress that you are listening. When it is your turn to speak, take the opportunity of confirming first of all that you have understood and enjoyed what the other person has said.

☐ At the end of a conversation, ask yourself how balanced it has been. Have you done all the talking? Or practically none of it? Do you feel you know much more about the other person than he or she knows about you, or vice versa? Ideally, you should balance your disclosures so that neither of you feels that the other is holding back. Nor should you feel that the other person is disclosing more personal information than you are prepared to give away about yourself.

☐ When you first meet someone, it is not a good idea to prolong the conversation longer than feels comfortable, or, if you are at a party or other social gathering, to cling to the person you have just met like a limpet. It is better to move on when things are still going well, leaving your new acquaintance free to meet other people. If you like him or her enough, say something that will make it obvious that you have enjoyed the conversation and would like to follow up the meeting ('It's been nice talking to you', 'Perhaps we'll meet again later').

Being sexually successful

Many men feel unhappy or frustrated because they consider themselves unsuccessful with women. This sense of failure is made worse by the fact that some men seem to have no difficulty at all in attracting any number of willing partners. But the most apparently successful men are not necessarily those who especially like women or have the best sex life. Their main pleasure is usually not derived from a caring and sharing sensuality, but from making sex into a competitive sport. Pleasure for these men is in the chase, or in being able to flaunt a beautiful new partner in public. It melts away once they have achieved their objective, so that they develop no real commitment to, or concern for, their partner and can move smoothly to the next port of call. To the onlooker, such easy promiscuity may seem enviable, but it is not a particularly satisfying way of life.

True sexual success depends on such things as self-esteem, assertiveness, the ability to relax, and a genuine liking and consideration for women. The following advice will help you move in this direction. Remember that however average or undistinguished you believe yourself to be, some women will have a preference for *you*, for the kind of person *you* are. If you are aware of this you will not always have to do all the pursuing.

What to do on the first date

It is usually best not to make the first date with a partner too 'heavy'. You may both be more comfortable if it is casual and informal – lunch or coffee during the day, for example, so that you can get to know each other without either of you wondering about what is going to happen afterward. Do not expect to be asked inside if you meet at her place, and do not turn up too early or late. Do not be stingy, but do not spend rashly either. Never fuss about the price when you are paying for a meal. If she offers to buy you a drink or to pay her way, accept. It will make the relationship more equal and let her

know that she has a choice about what you do. If you think she is offering out of politeness, do not accept immediately. If she really wants to pay, she will insist, and then you should let her.

Spend time and energy, as well as money, planning where to go and what to do. Try to picture the kind of things she might enjoy. Offer to cook for her, for example, and set the scene with soft lights, good music, comfortable and tidy surroundings. Find out what music she likes and get some suitable records or tapes. Or watch a good movie on TV together. If you go to a restaurant, choose one with atmosphere. But do not suggest anything that might make her feel uneasy on a first date. She might get worried, for example, if a picnic takes you to some very remote or deserted spot. Be flexible about meetings – if a last minute change of plan is unavoidable, or if she wants to cancel the date, be flexible about it. And never, when you are with her, show too much interest in other women you meet or see.

The importance of timing

Assuming that you continue meeting after the first date, the question will arise sooner or later of whether you are going to enter into a sexual relationship. The early stages of such a relationship are a game in which each of you makes moves to which the other responds, ideally with the situation developing at a pace which suits you both. A sense of timing is crucial, so that you can judge the right moment to accelerate the pace or to draw back a little and consolidate the position you hold.

If your timing is wrong it is probably because you have tried to act independently, either ignoring or misreading the signals your partner sends which tell you she is ready for the next move. Move too slowly and she is likely to become irritated or lose interest. Move too fast and you may put her under too much pressure. This may force her into a situation where she rejects you or backs away because she is not yet ready to go further and feels that this course is the only one you have left open to her.

Often, what you take to be a personal rejection by someone you have tried to date may simply be a matter of bad or unlucky timing. You may have chosen a time when she was involved with someone else, or caught her in the aftermath of a relationship when she needed to be free from involvement for a while to recover her emotional equilibrium. If you think there is a chance that this may be so, then do not be too discouraged. Keep your options open by maintaining casual contact with her and trying your luck again later. If you get the same message a second time, then accept defeat and move on.

Judging her response

Provided that your timing has been fortunate and that you are sending out the right signals through body language, you should be able to 'read' your partner's responses and judge when she is ready for you to step up the pace. Raised eyebrows, eyes wide open, and dilated pupils all indicate an encouraging response. If you find you are looking into each other's eyes for longer and longer periods, this is also a definite 'come-on' signal. Be appreciative if she stands close to you, or at least does not move away when you draw closer to her. You are getting a favorable response, too, if she nods her head in enthusiastic agreement with what you are saying, or occasionally touches you to emphasize a point she is making.

Do not take too much for granted

If your sexual advances are often rebuffed, it may be that you are assuming sex is your right, thereby reducing your partner's freedom of choice, so that rejection is likely, even inevitable. The following advice will help you to reassess your situation and probably to improve your success with prospective sexual partners.

☐ Do not look on every woman as a sex object or prize as soon as you meet her. The man who says, 'Your place or mine?' as soon as he has been introduced may win a few but he will lose many more.

☐ Do not assume that social responsiveness is the same as sexual encouragement. Because a woman is polite, or even friendly, this does not necessarily mean that she is ready to go to bed with you – or, at least, not yet. Look for definite signs of sexual interest before making a move.

☐ Do not expect every encounter, every date, to lead to sex. Keep your first dates casual so that you can get to know each other first.

☐ Do not be too familiar too soon. Show admiration in the way you look at her and interest in what she says and does. But unless you are very sure of your ground, do not use verbal endearments or physical caresses at a first meeting.

Sexual good manners

When it becomes clear that a sexual relationship is on the cards, remember that sensitivity plays as important a part in a new sexual encounter as it does at the beginning of any other relationship. By adopting the following advice you should avoid the worst breaches of sexual etiquette and so safeguard your developing relationship.

☐ Carry a packet of condoms with you so that if you find your partner is unprotected (you should always ask her whether she has any form of contraception) you can allay any fears of pregnancy.

☐ Make sure the sheets are clean if the venue is your bedroom. Reassure your partner if she has her period, that this need not prohibit sex as far as you are concerned, but do not press her if she prefers to wait until it is over. If she is willing, provide a clean towel for her to lie on.

☐ Suggest a bath, shower, or massage together first, especially if either of you is tense or nervous.

☐ Ask her how and where she likes to be touched and find out exactly what she wants to do. She may prefer to be the sexually active partner, or conversely, just to cuddle or sleep beside you the first time, rather than have sex.

☐ Do not in any circumstances resort to sexual blackmail by saying you love her if you do not or by making her feel that just because you are aroused she has an obligation to do something about it.

☐ Do not try so-called aphrodisiacs. They do not work and some are even dangerous. The most potent aphrodisiac of all is to be made to feel truly desirable. So tell your partner how much you admire and desire her and *never* criticize any imperfections in her looks or figure.

Your first sexual experience

Even if you are sexually experienced you may have problems at first with a new partner. You will be anxious to make a good impression, and may be so tense or nervous that you cannot get an erection, however much you want her. If you do get an erection you may lose it, or climax too soon through overexcitement. The situation may be very similar if it is your first ever sexual experience, except that in this case your problems will probably be compounded by the fact that your partner is equally inexperienced and nervous. Whatever happens, do not feel that you have failed if it is not quite as you hoped it would be, and do not take it too seriously, for the situation will improve as you gain confidence.

The following suggestions should help to make your sexual initiation more enjoyable.

☐ Never contemplate sex with a woman if you do not find her attractive.

☐ Make sure you have time, comfort, and privacy. Five minutes in the back of a car with an ever-present threat of discovery may rid you of your virginity, but it will not give you a true idea of how good sex can be.

☐ Do not be in too much of a hurry, especially if your partner is also sexually inexperienced. Make sure she is fully aroused, by caressing and stimulating her for at least ten minutes before you enter her. When she is fully aroused, her natural vaginal lubrication will make penetration easier. If she is tense because this is her first time too, it will probably be more comfortable for both of you if you use saliva or an artificial lubricant as well.

☐ Choose a man-on-top position (see SEXUAL POSITIONS, p.55) and put a pillow beneath your partner's hips so that it is easier to enter her. Spread her vaginal lips gently with your fingers and guide your penis between them.

☐ Push gently but firmly. You may need to apply some pressure if she is a virgin, but do not thrust hard. The hymen forms no real barrier since it is a very thin membrane that only partially covers the vaginal entrance. There will be very little pain and virtually no loss of blood when it is broken.

☐ Now begin to thrust lightly (but not deeply if it is her first time). Neither of you should feel let down if she does not reach orgasm; few women do the first few times they have sex and some rarely do, even with regular intercourse. For most women, being able to experience orgasm through intercourse is something that has to be learned and is not automatic as it is for men.

▽ **First intercourse**
The first time you have intercourse, it will probably be quite unlike what you imagined. But you should not take any disappointment too seriously, since you have plenty of time in which to learn the varied skills of lovemaking.

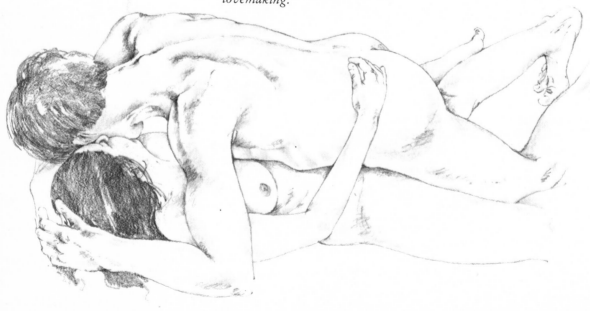

APPENDICES
SEX AND HEALTH

It is difficult for anyone to enjoy sex – and sometimes even to function sexually – if they are feeling ill or off-color. Any chronic or painful illness, for example, will almost always tend to decrease your capacity and desire for sex. If you are convalescing after an acute illness, you will probably find that your sexual appetite is reduced. Sometimes the drugs you have to take can affect sex drive and performance.

If your general life style is an unhealthy one, this too is often reflected in your sex-life. Heavy smoking and drinking can both lead to erection problems, for example. A serious weight problem means that in all probability you will be breathless, less mobile and therefore less sexually vigorous. Your mental state is important too. A depressive illness can affect your self-esteem and lower your sexual confidence. It is also likely to cause erection problems and a loss of sexual interest.

Some medical problems cause specific sexual difficulties – but often these are remediable. A few of the most common medical conditions that affect sexual functioning are discussed below. Your doctor may be able to give you further practical advice, and advise you about the side effects of particular drugs.

Diabetes mellitus
The condition can lead to erection problems, which are more severe the older you are and the longer you have the disease. You are less likely to develop the problem if the diabetes is treated by diet alone.

What you should do

Try not to dwell on the possibility – often if there is a problem it is mild, but worry may make it worse and can lead eventually to a loss of sexual interest.

Heart attack
Erection problems are quite common both immediately before and for some time after a heart attack, probably because the blood supply to the erectile tissue decreases. But the main problem is the anxiety that sex may bring on another attack.

What you should do

☐ Be reassured, if your doctor says it is alright to take moderate exercise, that sex will be safe.

☐ Get accustomed to masturbating once more before resuming sex with a partner.

☐ Keep your sexual encounters as stress-free as possible. New partners or illicit relationships may make you more anxious than a trusted partner in familiar surroundings.

☐ Take things easily at first, with occasional rest and no sexual gymnastics. After about 6 months your sexual activity should be back to normal.

Multiple sclerosis
Erection problems are common and sensation in the penis and the ability to ejaculate may be lost. However, in some cases increased sensitivity makes orgasm and even touch unpleasant.

What you should do

Use direct stimulation to produce an erection as this often works when fantasy does not.

Arthritis
Reduced mobility and the restriction of sexual activity are usually associated with this condition and others that cause stiff or painful joints.

What you should do

☐ Choose the time of day when you have least pain to make love.

☐ Take painkillers, if you use them, half an hour before making love.

☐ Before making love, rest and take a warm bath.

☐ Experiment to discover the most comfortable position. If movement is a problem, choose a position in which your partner can do most of the work. But if you cannot support her weight, use a rear-entry or side-by-side position (see SEXUAL POSITIONS, p.55).

Ileostomy/colostomy
Erection problems and, occasionally, ejaculatory difficulties or retrograde ejaculation (into the bladder) may follow these operations, especially in older men who have had the rectum removed.

Embarrassment about the condition and a fear of leakage may diminish sexual enjoyment.

What you should do

☐ Make quite sure that your bag fits well and securely.

☐ Learn to predict when your bag will be full and adjust your lovemaking accordingly. You will probably find it best, for example, not to make love for an hour or two after you have eaten.

☐ If the bag seems to get in the way, try a different position. It may seem less intrusive if your partner is on top, for example.

☐ Tell a new partner about your condition *before* you make love for the first time. Reassure her that sex will not harm the stoma (artificial orifice) or create any other medical problems.

☐ Until you are so accustomed to your bag that you can forget about it, you may feel more comfortable wearing something over it.

Spinal injuries

Erection may be impaired – the degree depends on the site and severity of the injury. But often it can be obtained by either physical or psychic (mental) stimulation. Ejaculation is often lost and fertility may be diminished in those men who can ejaculate.

What you should do

If you have a partial erection:

☐ Use any method that works to maintain it. If direct stimulation is used, make sure your partner realizes that she should continually stimulate your penis to maintain the erection.

☐ Experiment to discover the position in which an erection is most easily sustained. Often one in which the woman squats astride the man is the most suitable.

☐ With your partner's help you may be able to ease your penis into her. Then hold the base and move it around in her vagina.

If you have no erection:

☐ Remember that you and your partner can still make love using your hands and mouth (see STIMULATION TECHNIQUES p.50). You may discover that the sensitivity of other parts of your body, especially just above your genitals, seems to increase in a compensatory way.

☐ Artificial aids such as vibrators may be helpful. If you both like the idea, try an artificial penis. These are strapped to your body and are either solid or hollowed out so that your penis fits inside.

☐ In some cases mechanical aids may be used to support the penis. A semi-rigid rod insert produces a penis stiff enough for intercourse, but not permanently and entirely erect. When not 'in use' it can be bent down to hang in the normal way.

THE SEXUAL SIDE-EFFECTS OF DRUGS

Few drugs enhance sexual functioning, but many have adverse effects on it, and often on sex-drive as well. Anti-depressants may reduce sexual functioning, while anticonvulsants and antihypertensives reduce both sex drive and sexual functioning. 'Recreational' drugs, alcohol (in small doses), amphetamines, cocaine and marijuana, increase sexual desire, but nearly all – including tobacco – have an adverse effect on a person's ability to become aroused, enjoy sex and reach orgasm.

TESTING FOR AIDS

When someone is infected with the HIV virus that causes AIDS, their body develops antibodies against the virus. A blood test for the presence of HIV antibodies provides a fairly reliable indication as to whether or not the person is infected with the virus. If you are in a 'high risk' group, you may wonder whether to take the antibody test.

Testing does not prove that you will or will not develop AIDS. The test is not 100 per cent reliable; a second, different type of test is usually carried out on any positive sample to confirm the result. HIV antibodies take weeks (or even months) to develop, so a test taken shortly after you have been infected will give a negative result. A positive test shows that you have been exposed to the virus; it does not mean that you will inevitably develop AIDS.

People who are antibody positive are usually advised only to tell those who actually need to know – their doctor, dentist, close friends, and their sexual partner. Misconceptions about AIDS cause unnecessary discrimination against sufferers, or people who are antibody positive.

SEXUALLY TRANSMITTED DISEASES

Sexually transmitted diseases (also referred to as STD or, decreasingly, as venereal diseases or VD) are nearly always transferred from person to person through vaginal or anal intercourse or oral-genital contact. Most of the organisms that cause these diseases thrive only in warm, moist conditions and cannot survive outside the body for more than a few minutes. Therefore it is virtually impossible to contract an STD through contact with, say, a lavatory seat, although infection may occasionally be spread via a towel handled immediately after use by an infected person.

It is essential to seek medical help promptly either from your doctor or from a special clinic if you think you may have a sexually transmitted disease. Treatment is simple and effective provided it is started early enough. You should have no sexual relationships until you are cured, and it is important that your recent sexual partners contact a doctor immediately too, since during the incubation period you may have infected others.

Non-specific urethritis (NSU)

This is the most common sexually transmitted disease and 80 per cent of sufferers are male. About 45 per cent of cases are probably caused by a bacterium called chlamydia, but other microbes are also believed to cause the disease.

Symptoms Tingling in the tip of the penis, sometimes accompanied by a scant clear discharge. Both are most noticeable first thing in the morning and appear 1-5 weeks after the infection is contracted.

Treatment By antibiotics. Your partner should also be treated, even if she has no symptoms. You should not have sex until the treatment is complete.

Gonorrhea

One person in 100 develops gonorrhea (often called 'the clap') each year. It is more common in people who have many sexual partners, and two-thirds of sufferers are male. The disease is caused by a bacterium transmitted through vaginal or anal intercourse or oral sex.

Symptoms Discomfort in urination and a slight discharge of pus. Symptoms appear within 2-10 days of infection. Untreated, the disease may spread through the sexual organs, and obstruct the flow of urine. It can also lead to sterility. Anal infection may cause moistness and pain in the rectum; oral infection may result in mouth ulcers or a sore throat.

Treatment By antibiotics. You must abstain from sex until you are free of symptoms.

Genital herpes

A viral disease transmitted by direct body contact. Not everyone who comes into contact with herpes develops the disease, and many people have symptomless attacks and acquire immunity. The first bout of herpes may last 2-3 weeks. About half of all sufferers have subsequent attacks, but these tend to be shorter and less severe. Attacks tend to recur when the sufferer is physically run down or under stress.

Symptoms A genital rash of red patches with white, itching blisters which may burst to form shallow, painful ulcers. There may be tenderness and swelling in the groin, pain or a burning sensation during urination, fever, and general discomfort. Symptoms appear 2-20 days after contact.

Treatment There is at present no effective treatment, although a drug, acyclovir, reduces the period for which you are infectious. Acyclovir is most effective when treatment is started early in the attack; if you suffer frequent recurrences it is probably worth asking your doctor for a supply of the drug so that you can start to take it immediately you notice the early warning signs of tingling and numbness which usually develop a day or two before blisters appear. An analgesic such as aspirin or a local anaesthetic will reduce severe pain. Cold compresses and ice-packs ease discomfort, and painting the area with gentian violet may help. Wear cotton boxer-style briefs and avoid tight pants. Avoid intercourse from the moment the first tingling appears until the blisters have healed. Use condoms for about four weeks after the symptoms have vanished. A condom will protect your partner only if it covers the infected area.

Syphilis

Syphilis is rare. Most sufferers are male and most are homosexual. The disease organism usually enters through the urethra, rectum or mouth.

Symptoms The first sign is a hard, painless, highly infectious sore on the penis and anus. It takes 9-90 days to appear and disappears spontaneously after a few weeks. The disease can be successfully treated with antibiotics; if untreated, a non-irritant rash, and swollen lymph glands, may develop some weeks later. Warty lumps may appear around the anus if it was the site of original infection. The disease then enters a symptom-free stage. More serious symptoms, leading eventually to death, may develop years later.

Genital warts

These appear as small cauliflower-like growths on the genitals or around the anus. They are caused by a virus that is transmitted by direct body contact, and appear between one and six months after the infection.

Treatment Application of a caustic substance, or by freezing or electrical cauterization.

Pubic lice ('crabs')

Minute blood-sucking insects which appear in the pubic or anal hair. The lice appear several weeks after the infection and may cause severe itching, especially at night.

Treatment Application of a special cream or lotion.

GUIDELINES FOR SAFER SEX

Sex does not cause AIDS. Being frightened of the disease does not mean you have to give up sex, nor does it mean avoiding physical contact with an infected person. It is safe to live with someone who has AIDS, to sleep in the same bed, share the same household utensils, and hug them. The danger lies in allowing an infected person's body fluids – blood, semen, vaginal fluids and (to a much lesser extent) saliva to enter your own body through a cut or an abrasion.

The table below puts various sexual activities into categories according to the risk they involve. It is important to realise that in our present state of knowledge it is impossible to say with absolute certainty exactly how risky any form of sex is. The virus has been found in saliva, for example, and although there is no evidence as yet that AIDS has ever been acquired by kissing, one can't say with certainty that this is impossible. We can, however, say that it is unlikely. So it is that on a balance of possibilities – erring on the cautious side – that the risks of various sexual activities have been assessed.

In general, 'safer sex' means using a barrier during sexual activities which involve an exchange of body fluids, or avoiding those activities altogether. The HIV virus cannot penetrate the latex of which condoms are made, so using latex as a barrier between you and your partner's body fluids is an effective safety measure. Condoms should be used during intercourse (extra-strong ones during anal intercourse). Nonoxynol-9, an ingredient of most spermicides, kills the HIV virus, so use spermicide as well as a condom as an additional safety measure. Alternatively, buy a brand of condom which is itself lubricated with nonoxynol-9.

If you are infected yourself, 'safe sex' precautions are still sensible even if your only sexual partner is another infected person. A characteristic of the HIV virus is that it constantly changes its structure within the body. Someone who is re-infected with a variation of the virus may develop a new and different set of symptoms.

Monogamy is the best guarantee of a really safe sex life. If you change partners often, or if your regular partner has other sexual contacts, the only sensible policy is always to use a condom and spermicide whenever you have intercourse.

NO RISK
Solo and mutual masturbation; body massage (excluding the genital area); using unshared sex toys (e.g. vibrators, dildoes).

LOW RISK
Intercourse (anal or vaginal) with a condom and spermicide; fellatio ("sucking") without ejaculation, or wearing a condom; anilingus ("rimming") i.e. oral-anal sex, through a latex barrier.

HIGH RISK
Anal and vaginal intercourse without a condom; "Fisting" – insertion of the hand into the rectum (the risk is lessened if a latex glove is worn); using shared sex toys; any sex act which draws blood.

AIDS

AIDS – Acquired Immune Deficiency Syndrome – is caused by the human immunodeficiency virus (HIV). The virus is present in body fluids – blood, semen, and sometimes saliva, though in saliva the quantities are probably too small to cause infection. AIDS is primarily a sexually transmitted disease, but it can also be passed on by transfusion with infected blood, or by the shared use of a hypodermic needle or syringe among intravenous drug users.

Once inside the body, the virus penetrates and multiplies inside the T4 white blood cells which play a vital part in the body's defences against some infections and cancers. Eventually the cells burst, releasing HIV particles into the blood which can then infect more T4 blood cells. As cells are gradually destroyed, the person becomes more prone to infections of the lungs, gut, or brain, or to various forms of cancer, such as Kaposi's sarcoma, a rare form of skin cancer. At the moment it seems probable that between 1 in 10 and 1 in 3 of those infected with the virus will eventually develop AIDS.

AIDS cannot be transmitted by casual social contact; to cause infection, the virus must actually enter the body through a cut or abrasion in the skin or the mucous membranes which line the rectum, vagina or mouth. The rectum is especially vulnerable because its lining is thin and delicate, so anal intercourse carries a higher risk than most other forms of sexual activity. However, the disease can also be spread by vaginal intercourse. Use of a condom helps to prevent infection (see **Guidelines for safer sex**, p.154). Most doctors believe that the chances of catching AIDS from a single sexual encounter with an infected person are very small. It is repeated sexual contact with an infected person or persons that is likely to lead to infection. The HIV virus cannot survive for long outside the body, and is destroyed by ordinary household bleaches and disinfectants, or by detergent diluted in hot water. If the blood of an infected person is spilt, it can be safely cleaned up using any of these. Unless the infected blood actually enters your own bloodstream through some skin lesion it cannot harm you.

Symptoms Some people infected with the HIV virus do not develop symptoms, though they can still infect others. A few people develop a mononucleosis-like illness soon after infection, which clears up without treatment, but most feel perfectly well. People who have had the infection for some months or years may develop permanently swollen lymph glands, and tend to develop common skin infections. Some people go on to develop a variety of symptoms, including fever, weight loss, diarrhea and oral thrush, which are known as the AIDS-related complex, or ARC. ARC is not itself fatal, but people who develop it are more likely to develop full-blown AIDS. This usually has a pattern of repeated infections, weight loss, weakness and eventual death. On average, about 3-4 years elapse between infection and the development of AIDS.

Treatment Although there is no vaccine or cure for AIDS at present, the conditions associated with it can often be treated. Early trials suggest that in a few cases the drug Retrovir (AZT) may 'buy time' by slowing down the progress of the disease, though the drug has very unpleasant side-effects.

Hepatitis B

Hepatitis B is an infection of the liver which is most common in tropical countries. It is caused by a virus which, like the AIDS virus, is transmitted through contact with infected blood, usually by the shared use of needles by drug users, blood transfusion, and sexual contact. The disease can also be passed from an infected woman to her baby during pregnancy.

Symptoms Jaundice, weakness, loss of appetite, nausea and abdominal discomfort are the most common symptoms. They may be severe and last for some weeks. In a few people the disease causes chronic liver damage. Some of those who have been infected may continue to carry the virus and transmit it to others even though they have no symptoms themselves. A blood test will determine whether or not you are a symptomless carrier.

Treatment It is now possible to be vaccinated against hepatitis B; if you frequently travel abroad or have a sex life which puts you particularly at risk, vaccination is a sensible precaution.

RESOURCE GUIDE

RECOMMENDED READING

General

Bancroft, J. *Human Sexuality and Its Problems* (2nd edition). London: Churchill Livingstone, 1989.

Barbach, L. *For Each Other: Sharing Sexual Intimacy*. New York: Doubleday, 1982.

Comfort, A. *The Joy of Sex*. New York: Simon and Schuster, 1974.

Friday, N. *Men in Love: Male Sexual Fantasies*. New York: Dell, 1983.

Gochros, J. L. and J. Fischer. *Treat Yourself to a Better Sex Life*. Englewood Cliffs, NJ: Prentice-Hall, 1980.

Kubler-Ross, E. *AIDS: The Ultimate Challenge*. New York: Macmillan, 1988.

Lacroix, N. *Sensual Massage*. New York: Henry Holt, 1990.

Nowinski, J. *Becoming Satisfied: A Man's Guide to Good Sex*. New York: Warner, 1984.

McCarthy, B. and E. McCarthy. *Male Sexual Awareness: Enhancing Sexual Pleasure*. New York: Carroll & Graf, 1988.

Westheimer, W. *Dr. Ruth's Guide to Good Sex*. New York: Warner, 1984.

Zilbergeld, B. *Male Sexuality*. New York: Warner, 1984.

For older readers

Butler, R. N. and M. I. Lewis. *Love and Sex After Sixty: A Guide for Men and Women in Their Later Years*. New York: Harper & Row, 1976.

Gershenfeld, M. *How to Find Love, Sex and Intimacy*. New York: Fawcett, 1991.

For disabled or handicapped readers

Comfort, A. *Sexual Consequences of Disability*. Philadelphia: Lippincott, 1978.

Mooney, T., T. Cole and R. Chilgren. *Sexual Options for Paraplegics and Quadriplegics*. Boston: Little, Brown, 1975.

ORGANIZATIONS

Advice on sexual issues and related problems

American Association of Sex Educators, Counselors, and Therapists (AASECT)
435 N. Michigan Avenue
Suite 1717
Chicago, IL 60611
(312) 644-0828

Sex Information and Education Council of the U.S., Resources Center and Library
130 W. 42nd Street
Suite 2500
New York, NY 10036
(212) 819-9770

Information services for homosexuals or those with sexual orientation concerns

Div. 44, Gay and Lesbian Concerns, American Psychological Association
1200 17th Street NW
Washington, DC 20036
(202) 955-7600

Institute for Human Identity
118 W. 72nd Street
New York, NY 10023
(212) 799-9432

Los Angeles Gay and Lesbian Community Services Center
1213 N. Highland Avenue
Los Angeles, CA 90038
(213) 464-7400

Information on sexually transmitted diseases (STDs)

Clinics are listed in your local telephone directories, usually under the heading Social and Human Services. For information about STDs, contact the following services.

National sexually transmitted disease hotline
(800) 227-8922

National herpes hotline
(919) 361-8488

HIV/AIDS information service
(800) 342-2437

Index

Your Sexual Profile Chart

Use the chart below to create your own sexual profile. See p.20 for instructions.

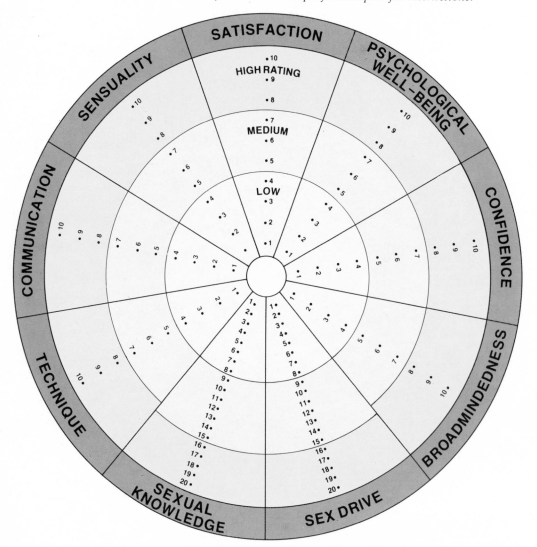

KEY TO ORIENTATION QUESTIONNAIRE (p.19)

☐ **A** You are exclusively heterosexual.

☐ **B** You are predominantly heterosexual, but under some conditions you may show a flicker of homosexual interest.

☐ **C** You are predominantly heterosexual, but have a strong element of homosexuality.

☐ **D** You are bisexual.

☐ **E** You are predominantly homosexual, but have an element of heterosexuality.

☐ **F** You are predominantly homosexual.

☐ **G** You are exclusively homosexual.